Practical Cardiology for Veterinary Nurses

This concise textbook provides a comprehensive, practical guide for veterinary nurses and technicians who wish to develop their knowledge, confidence, and skills when nursing the cardiac patient. Presentation of dogs or cats with heart disease is common, and it is vital that nurses understand how to look after these patients appropriately and support owners through what can often be challenging times. The book:

- Begins with basic anatomy and physiology, foundations required to understand the disease processes explained in later chapters
- Covers diseases seen in small animal practice, including congenital disease, heart failure, and treatment options
- Gives the nurse a sound understanding of electrocardiography, thoracic radiography, and cardiac ultrasound – how to perform these, and of what they are seeing
- Covers the hands-on requirements of the veterinary nurse, such as heart auscultation and feeling patient pulses
- Lists cardiac drugs, explaining when and why pharmacology would be used, as well as side effects
- Has a dedicated chapter on first aid
- Discusses chronic nursing management of heart conditions, including remote monitoring, support, and care planning

The book is packed with learning features including a glossary, diagrams, illustrations and tables in full colour, concise end of chapter key points, and further reading lists. Essential reading for student nurses and technicians, as well as those in practice who need a quick reference 'on the ground', this is the book that general practice veterinary nurses have been waiting for.

"I am so excited to see a book like this be released. Charlotte Pace has brought together a fantastic pocket-sized resource for veterinary nurses and technicians interested in learning about Cardiology. Her expert insight and knowledge has ensured this book is jam packed with all the information and quick reference guides that nurses and technicians would require for the day to day nursing of cardiac patients. I really wish this was about at the start of my cardiology journey —I would have had to get two, as the one in my pouch would have been completely battered with use!"

Sara-Ann Dickson BSc, RVN, VTS (IM - Cardiology), AFHEA,
Cardiology Nurse, UK

Practical Cardiology for Veterinary Nurses

Charlotte Pace

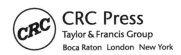

CRC Press
Taylor & Francis Group
Boca Raton London New York

CRC Press is an imprint of the
Taylor & Francis Group, an **informa** business

First edition published 2023
by CRC Press
6000 Broken Sound Parkway NW, Suite 300, Boca Raton, FL 33487-2742

and by CRC Press
4 Park Square, Milton Park, Abingdon, Oxon, OX14 4RN

CRC Press is an imprint of Taylor & Francis Group, LLC

© 2023 Taylor & Francis Group, LLC

ISBN: 978-0-367-64106-1 (hbk)
ISBN: 978-0-367-64102-3 (pbk)
ISBN: 978-1-003-12217-3 (ebk)

DOI: 10.1201/9781003122173

Typeset in Minion
by KnowledgeWorks Global Ltd.

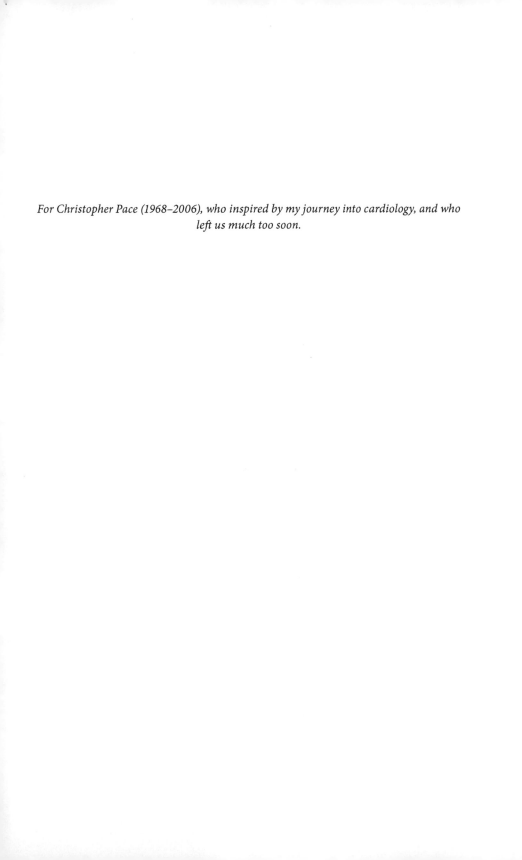

For Christopher Pace (1968–2006), who inspired by my journey into cardiology, and who left us much too soon.

Contents

List of figures, tables and boxes   ix

Acknowledgements   xv

About the author   xvii

Introduction   1
1 Structure and function of the heart   3
2 Acquired heart disease in dogs   15
3 Acquired heart disease in cats   33
4 Congenital heart disease   49
5 Electrocardiography   59
6 The nurse's role in diagnostic tests   83
7 Drugs   105
8 Cardiac emergencies – First aid   119

Glossary   131

Index   139

List of figures, tables and boxes

FIGURES

1.1	Diagram of the thorax showing position of the lobar divisions	4
1.2	Diagram of three layers of the heart wall	4
1.3	Diagram of the four chambers with valves labelled and great arteries shown	5
1.4	Diagram showing intracardiac systolic and diastolic pressures	5
1.5	Diagram showing pattern of blood flow, using red and blue to denote the difference in oxygenated and deoxygenated blood	7
1.6	Diagram of conduction system labelled, marking the left and right bundles	7
1.7	Cycle of compensated heart failure	10
1.8	Cycle of decompensated heart failure	11
2.1	Diagram of labelled mitral valve	17
2.2	Mitral valve regurgitation seen on echocardiography	17
2.3	Picture of dog with ascites	19
2.4	Echocardiographic image of a normal canine heart	21
2.5	Echocardiographic image of MMVD at stage B2	21
2.6	Echocardiographic image of MMVD at stage C	22
2.7	Example of cachexia in a dog	24
2.8	DCM seen on echocardiography	27
2.9	Dog wearing a 24-hour Holter ECG monitor	29
3.1	Normal cat heart on echocardiography, in right parasternal axis view	35
3.2	Normal cat heart on echocardiography in a different view (short axis), showing the left atrium (LA) to aorta (Ao) ratio	35
3.3	HCM on echocardiography, in right parasternal axis view	36
3.4	HCM on echocardiography showing the left atrium (LA) to aorta ratio (Ao) in short axis	36
3.5	Echocardiographic picture of extremely large left atrium (LA) compared to the aorta (AO)	37
3.6	Echocardiographic picture of thrombus in left atrium (LA)	37
3.7	Cat with an ATE affecting one limb	39
3.8	Diagram of SAM	40
3.9	Thoracentesis in a cat	44
3.10	Image of B Lines on ultrasound	46
4.1	Picture of a VSD	50
4.2	VSD on echo	50
4.3	Picture of a PDA	51
4.4	PDA seen on echocardiography	51

4.5	An Amplatz canine ductal occluder	52
4.6	Picture of AS	53
4.7	Picture of PS	54
4.8	(a) Fluoroscopy image showing balloon catheter across the pulmonic valve. The waist indicates the stenosis. And (b) fluoroscopy image showing the waist has gone	55
4.9	Picture of Tetralogy of Fallot	56
4.10	Part of ToF visible on echocardiography	56
5.1	Picture of digital ECG machine with electrodes and cables	60
5.2	Picture of electrodes	61
5.3	Gold standard positioning for an ECG	62
5.4	How the ECG leads form a triangle around the heart and become a three lead trace	62
5.5	How three leads become six leads on an ECG trace, using different viewpoints	63
5.6	This is a six lead ECG trace	63
5.7	Artefact in leads I and II, caused by movement. Red circles highlight interference	65
5.8	Purring artefact	65
5.9	Labelled diagram of the conduction system	68
5.10	Labelled diagram of a sinus complex	68
5.11	Shows ECG ruler measuring 25 mm/second	69
5.12	Shows ECG ruler measuring 50 mm/second	70
5.13	Following this simple heart rate algorithm can help narrow down arrhythmia possibilities	71
5.14	Summary of Questions 2–4	72
5.15	Example of a wide and bizarre complex in an otherwise sinus rhythm	72
5.16	Example of tall and narrow complex in an otherwise sinus rhythm	73
5.17	Example of left anterior fascicular block in a cat	73
5.18	Sinus rhythm in a dog	73
5.19	Sinus rhythm in a cat	74
5.20	Sinus tachycardia in a dog. Heart rate is 180 beats/minute	74
5.21	Sinus bradycardia in a cat. Heart rate is 80 beats/minute	74
5.22	Sinus arrhythmia	74
5.23	Atrial fibrillation. Heart rate is 229 beats/minute	76
5.24	Ventricular tachycardia	77
5.25	Example of 2nd degree AV block. Heart rate is 86 beats/minute. This example is Mobitz type I because the P-R interval changes on the trace. Arrows denote unconducted P waves	78
5.26	Example of third degree Av block in a dog	78
5.27	Example of third degree AV block in a cat. Heart rate is 40 beats/minute	79
5.28	Atrial standstill. Heart rate is 40 beats/minute	79
5.29	Progression of an arrhythmia to ventricular fibrillation. The trace starts with sinus rhythm with occasional VPCs, progresses to ventricular tachycardia and ultimately ventricular fibrillation	80

6.1	Picture of stethoscope labelled	84
6.2	Auscultation of the heart base for the pulmonic and aortic valves, on the left hand side of the thorax	85
6.3	Auscultation of the sternum in cats	85
6.4	Auscultation of the mitral valve, at the apex of the heart on the right hand side of the thorax	86
6.5	Auscultation of the tricuspid valve, at the apex of the heart on the right hand side of the thorax	87
6.6	Auscultation whilst palpating pulses, such as the femoral artery, can help identify pulse deficits	87
6.7	Diagram showing when a systolic heart murmur sound can be heard in the cardiac cycle	89
6.8	Dog with pronounced temporal muscle wastage	90
6.9	Dog with cardiac cachexia. It has a prominent spine and poor coat condition	91
6.10	Example of normal mucous membrane colour	92
6.11	Equipment prepared and ready for use in cat	94
6.12	Placement of ultrasound probe on a dog	95
6.13	Blood pressure in a cat	95
6.14	Blood pressure in a dog. Both the cat and dog blood pressure measurements were taken in the consult room so the patient did not have to see other dogs or cats	96
6.15	Tips to stress free venepuncture	97
6.16	Photograph of jugular blood sampling	97
6.17	Photograph of sampling a lateral saphenous vein	97
6.18	Positioning for lateral thoracic radiographs	98
6.19	Positioning for DV thoracic radiographs. A sandbag was added across the neck at the last minute to minimise stress	99
6.20	Canine DV thoracic radiograph of a healthy dog	99
6.21	Canine lateral thoracic radiograph of a healthy dog	100
6.22	Canine lateral thoracic radiograph of a dog with severe heart failure	100
6.23	Canine DV thoracic radiograph of a dog with severe heart failure	101
6.24	Patient prepared for echocardiography, lying in right lateral recumbency	102
7.1	Diagram of kidney nephron showing the where different diuretics act	106
7.2	Diagram showing where neurohormonal drugs work in the renin-angiotensin-aldosterone system	108
7.3	Action potential of a working myocardial cell	112
8.1	Equipment needed for thoracocentesis. A box could be used with equipment prepared, and a checklist	122
8.2	Photograph showing gentle restraint of a cat about to undergo thoracocentesis	123
8.3	Preparation before thoracocentesis procedure	123
8.4	Syringe, butterfly catheter and three way tap	124
8.5	Thoracocentesis being performed and pleural fluid being removed	125

8.6   Equipment needed for pericardiocentesis   125
8.7   Collapsed patient receiving supplemental oxygen via mask   127
8.8   Machine capable of defibrillation (paddles on top), temporary pacing using
       transthoracic adhesive pads, and electrical cardioversion to convert atrial
       fibrillation to sinus rhythm   128

TABLES

1.1   Actions of the compensatory mechanisms   9
1.2   Summary of the effects of angiotensin II   9
1.3   Clinical signs associated with congestive heart failure   11
1.4   Clinical signs associated with forward heart failure   12
2.1   Compensatory mechanisms activated in when cardiac output is
       compromised   18
2.2   Classification of MMVD   20
2.3   Breeds with a high prevalence of DCM   26
2.4   Stages of DCM   27
3.1   Description of phenotypic groups in feline cardiology   34
3.2   Results of one study of 250 cats assessing limbs affected by aortic
       thromboembolism   38
3.3   Clinical signs of feline heart disease   38
3.4   Clinical signs of a thrombotic event   38
3.5   Findings of a study investigating the prevalence of heart murmurs and
       heart disease in healthy cats   40
3.6   Summary of the feline classification system   41
4.1   Most common CHD reported in dogs and cats in order of prevalence   50
5.1   Terminology   60
5.2   Electrode placement   61
5.3   Component parts of the sinus complex   64
5.4   Expected heart rates   69
5.5   Possible answers for Question 2   70
5.6   Possible answers for Question 3   71
5.7   Possible answers for Question 4   71
6.1   Summary to maximise auscultation technique   88
6.2   Causes of heart murmurs   89
7.1   Summary of diuretics   106
7.2   Summary of positive inotropes and doses   107
7.3   Summary of neurohormonal blockers and doses   108
7.4   Summary of medications used in the treatment of feline heart disease,
       ATE, and heart failure   111
7.5   Types of myocyte   112
7.6   Vaughan-Williams classification of anti-arrhythmic drugs   113
7.7   Drugs used in the management of bradyarrhythmias   116
8.1   Presentation and emergency treatment   121
8.2   Summary of treatment for arrhythmias   128

BOXES

2.1 Alternative names to describe mitral valve disease 16
2.2 Breeds predisposed to MMVD 16
2.3 Clinical signs of heart failure resulting from MMVD 19
2.4 Clinical signs of DCM 28
3.1 Breeds predisposed to HCM 34
5.1 How to ensure a good ECG trace is recorded 66
5.2 Common causes of arrhythmias 75
6.1 Heart sounds 83
6.2 Assessing pulse quality 91
6.3 Mucous membrane colour seen in cardiac patients 91
6.4 Blood pressure equipment list 93
7.1 Treatment when a cat has presented with a thrombus 110
8.1 Auscultation and physical findings in a cardiac emergency 120

Acknowledgements

Thanks to Dave Dickson, BVetMed, DVC, MRCVS, at Heart Vets and Paul Smith, BVetMed, DVC, MRCVS, from East Anglia Cardiology.

About the author

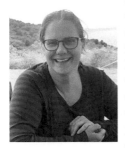

Charlotte Pace qualified as a veterinary nurse in 2003, whilst working in practice in London. In the same year she moved to the Royal Veterinary College to work as a medicine nurse. In 2006, she became the dedicated cardiology nurse for the Queen Mother Hospital for Animals. In 2010, she passed American veterinary technician exams and became the first nurse to hold the Cardiology qualification outside the US. From 2012 to 2015, Charlotte taught veterinary nurses on both degree and diploma programmes. In 2015, she returned to veterinary practice. She is a visiting lecturer and continues to write and lecture on veterinary cardiology. She is an active clinical coach and a member of the editorial board for *The Veterinary Nurse*, a position she has held since 2012. She is a member of the BVNA council and will be President in the year 2022–2023.

Introduction

It has been reported that around 10% of dogs in general practice have a diagnosis of heart disease[1], and it is estimated that approximately 15% of the cat population are affected by cardiac disease[2]. Recent data suggests that almost a third of cats over the age of nine years, have hypertrophic cardiomyopathy, whilst nearly two thirds of cats will have a heart murmur at this age[3]. Despite these figures showing the relatively common occurrence of heart disease in small animals, there is little focus on cardiology in the veterinary nursing syllabus and in general nursing textbooks.

The aim of this book is to provide a comprehensive, practical guide for veterinary nurses who wish to develop their knowledge, confidence and skills when nursing the cardiac patient. It is suitable for both student and qualified nurses. Presentation of dogs or cats with heart disease varies from asymptomatic to life threatening heart failure, or in cats, with additional complications such as arterial thromboembolism. It is vital that nurses understand how to look after these patients appropriately, to provide optimal care when nursing dyspnoeic and difficult patients, and support owners through what can often be challenging times.

Chapter 1 covers the basic structure of the heart, function, and normal pressures, and explains how heart disease occurs, and how heart failure can develop. The mechanisms of heart failure are explained to help nursing care of both the patient in acute, life threatening heart failure, and the chronic management of cases. Chapter 2 focuses on the most commonly acquired cardiac diseases in dogs. It starts with mitral valve disease, which accounts for about 75% of dogs diagnosed with acquired heart disease[1]. It also looks at dilated cardiomyopathy, the second most common acquired disease. This chapter will help nurses understand the pathophysiology, classification systems, presenting signs and the diagnostic tests used. This chapter also looks at the different treatment options and medications given, and prognosis, with special emphasis on the nurses' role in caring for these patients.

Chapter 3 looks at the same issues in feline disease, focusing on the different phenotypes identified in feline cardiac disease. Hypertrophic cardiomyopathy is the most prevalent, but other types that might be encountered are also described. This chapter will also look at appropriate cat handling techniques to maximise nursing skills, working with cats that may be frightened and/or dyspnoeic.

Chapter 4 examines the pathophysiology of congenital cardiac diseases seen in canine and feline populations, with specific reference to how they may present in practice. Treatment options are also discussed, including surgery, non-interventional techniques, and medical management.

Chapter 5 focuses on electrocardiography (ECGs). This chapter is particularly of use to nurses who want to learn how to use their ECG machine and to be able to use it confidently in any situation. The chapter shows how to set up the machine, use optimal

DOI: 10.1201/9781003122173-1

settings, and how to produce a trustworthy and reliable trace. It explores commonly seen problems when using the machine. It also looks at common arrhythmias, possible causes and treatment options, and appropriate nursing care.

Chapter 6 looks at the broader subject of diagnostic tests and the cardiac patient, including auscultation, physical examination, measuring blood pressure, blood sampling, radiography, and echocardiography. Discussion is focused on achieving reliable and repeatable results whilst minimising stress.

Chapter 7 discusses drugs used in the treatment of heart disease, heart failure, management of aortic thromboembolism, and the treatment of arrhythmias. Dose rates are provided, along with adverse reactions and nursing instructions for monitoring. Chapter 8 outlines emergency first aid treatment of patients presenting in respiratory distress, collapse, and/or with a thrombus. Kit lists are provided for thoracocentesis and pericardiocentesis, along with a protocol for nurses to follow. A glossary is included at the end of the book.

REFERENCES

1. Keene BW, Atkins CE, Bonagura JD, Fox PR, Häggström J, Fuentes VL, Oyama MA, Rush JE, Stepien R, Uechi M (2019). ACVIM consensus guidelines for the diagnosis and treatment of myxomatous mitral valve disease in dogs. *Journal of Veterinary Internal Medicine.* 33(3): 1127–1140

2. Payne JR, Brodbelt DC, Luis Fuentes V (2015). Cardiomyopathy prevalence in 780 apparently healthy cats in rehoming centres (the CatScan study). *Journal of Veterinary Cardiology.* 17 Suppl 1: S244–S257

3. Luis Fuentes V, Abbott J, Chetboul V, Côté E, Fox PR, Häggström J, Kittleson MD, Schober K, Stern JA (2020). ACVIM consensus statement guidelines for the classification, diagnosis, and management of cardiomyopathies in cats. *Journal of Veterinary Internal Medicine.* 34: 1062–1077.

Structure and function of the heart

The heart is a muscular organ that works by electrical stimulus. It has a crucial role in delivering oxygen and nutrients around the body and maintaining blood pressure. It is located in the thoracic cavity, within the mediastinum and in the pericardium. It lies between the third and sixth ribs, slightly to the left of the midline. Figure 1.1 shows the location of the heart in the thorax. The pericardium consists of a double layer of serous membrane. The outer layer is known as the parietal pericardium, and the inner layer is the visceral pericardium.

HEART WALL

The heart wall consists of three layers, shown in Figure 1.2:

- *Epicardium or serous pericardium* – This is the outer layer which produces serous fluid to lubricate the pericardial cavity.
- *Myocardium* – The middle layer. It is the largest part of the heart wall and is responsible for the pumping action. Blood is supplied to it by the coronary arteries.
- *Endocardium* – The inner layer. It consists of endothelial cells and creates a continuous lining with the wall and valves.

HEART VALVES

The heart has two sets of valves, two atrioventricular valves and two semilunar valves. The atrioventricular valves close at the onset of systole, as the ventricles contract. The semilunar valves close at the onset of diastole, as the ventricles relax. The valves all open one way only, to prevent blood from flowing in the wrong direction.

ATRIOVENTRICULAR VALVES

Mitral valve – Located between the left atrium and left ventricle, and has two cusps, or leaflets. Other names include the bicuspid valve or the left atrioventricular valve.

Tricuspid valve – Located between the right atrium and right ventricle, and has three cusps, or leaflets. Other names include the right atrioventricular valve.

The atrioventricular valves are attached to papillary muscles in the endocardium by tendons called chordae tendineae. These chordae tendineae are like hinges that prevent the valves from springing backwards.

DOI: 10.1201/9781003122173-2

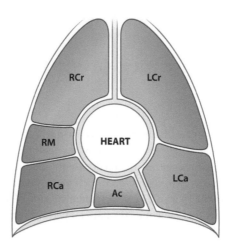

Figure 1.1 Diagram of the thorax showing position of the lobar divisions. Ac = Accessory lobe. LCa = Left caudal lobe. LCr = Left cranial lobe. RCa = Right caudal lobe. RCr = Right cranial lobe. RM = Right middle lobe.

SEMILUNAR VALVES

Aortic valve – Located at the bottom of the aorta. It has three cusps, or leaflets in a semilunar shape.

Pulmonic valve – Located at the bottom of the pulmonary artery. It also has three cusps, or leaflets in a semilunar shape.

CHAMBERS OF THE HEART

The heart consists of four sections, two upper chambers, the left and right atrium (*pleural atria*), and the left and right ventricles. The left and right sides of the heart are divided by a

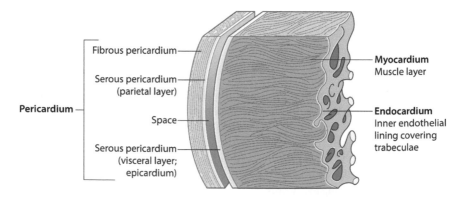

Figure 1.2 Diagram of three layers of the heart wall.

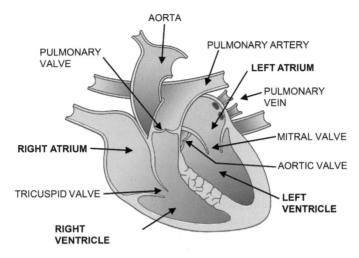

Figure 1.3 Diagram of the four chambers with valves labelled and great arteries shown.

septal wall. In the atria, this is called the atrial septum, and in the ventricles, the ventricular septum. The atria are smaller chambers and have thinner walls than the ventricles. Figure 1.3 shows the different chambers, with the heart valves and great arteries. Each chamber has a different function; therefore, each chamber has a different intracardiac pressure. Figure 1.4 summarises the systolic and diastolic pressures of the chambers and great arteries.

Left atrium – Collecting chamber for oxygenated blood. Systolic pressure less than 10 mmHg.

Left ventricle – The main chamber that provides oxygenated blood to the body. It is three times thicker than the right ventricle and operates at an approximate average of systolic 150 mmHg.

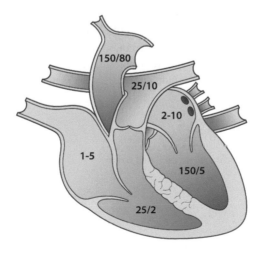

Figure 1.4 Diagram showing intracardiac systolic and diastolic pressures.

Right atrium – Collecting chamber for deoxygenated blood. Systolic pressure less than 5 mmHg.

Right ventricle – Chamber that provides deoxygenated blood to the lungs. It does not need to operate at the same high pressures as the left ventricle and works at an average pressure of 25 mmHg systolic.

> • *Systole* – Contraction of both ventricles, after the atrioventricular valves (mitral and tricuspid) have closed, ejecting blood into the aorta and pulmonary artery
> • *Diastole* – Relaxation of both ventricles, after semilunar (aortic and pulmonic) valves have closed, allowing blood to fill the ventricles

Knowing the intracardiac pressures of the individual chambers helps understand what happens when the heart becomes diseased. Any disease process on the left side of the heart will show clinical signs sooner than the equivalent on the right. Due to the lower pressures on the right side of the heart, the disease process must be moderate to severe to exhibit clinical signs, whereas relatively mild changes on the left can cause clinical signs. When the heart is diseased, higher intracardiac pressures can occur. This can be due to excessive fluid volume, as seen with heart congestive heart failure (CHF), or diseases that affect the contraction or relaxation of the ventricles (such as hypertrophic or dilated cardiomyopathy), or a narrowing or obstruction of the great arteries or chambers.

PATHWAY OF BLOOD

Oxygenated blood enters the left atrium via four pulmonary veins. Oxygenated blood passes from the left atrium across the mitral valve and into the left ventricle. The atrium contracts or squeezes the remaining blood to maximise efficiency. The one-way mitral valve then closes, to prevent blood from flowing backwards, and blood is pumped out of the left ventricle into the aorta and around the body. At the same time as the left side of the heart, deoxygenated blood enters the right atrium via the inferior and superior vena cava. Blood flows across the tricuspid valve, helped by an atrial contraction to optimise function. The tricuspid valve closes at the same time as the mitral valve, to prevent backflow, and as the ventricle contracts, blood is pushed to the lungs via the pulmonary artery. See Figure 1.5 for pathways of blood.

THE CARDIAC CYCLE

Events of the cardiac cycle are summarised below.

Systole	Diastole
Mitral and tricuspid valves close	Aortic and pulmonic valves close
Aorta and pulmonary valves open	Mitral and tricuspid valves open
Ventricles contract and blood is pumped out	Ventricles relax
	Atria contract

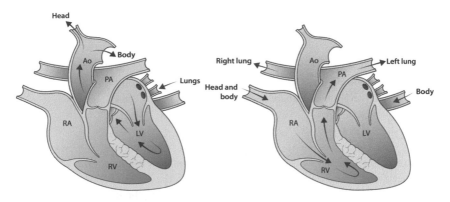

Figure 1.5 Diagram showing pattern of blood flow, using red and blue to denote the difference in oxygenated and deoxygenated blood.

CONDUCTION SYSTEM OF THE HEART

The cardiac conduction system is a network of specialised conduction cells that initiate and coordinate the contraction of the heart. Figure 1.6 shows the location of each section of the conduction system. The main features are as follows:

SINOATRIAL NODE (SA NODE)

The SA node is known as the pacemaker of the conduction system because it initiates an electrical impulse which travels across the atrium, depolarising the atrial myocardium as it goes. It is located in the right atrium.

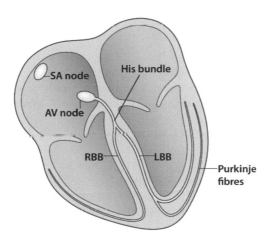

Figure 1.6 Diagram of conduction system labelled, marking the left and right bundles.

ATRIOVENTRICULAR NODE (AV NODE)

The AV node lies at the top of the atrioventricular septum. When the electrical impulse has depolarised the atria, it arrives at the AV node and passes through to the ventricles. Conduction is forced through the AV node because of a fibrous ring that prevents the impulse from travelling anywhere else except the specialised cells.

BUNDLE OF HIS

The Bundle of His are specialised cells within the intraventricular septum. The early part of the electrical impulse passes from the AV node to the left bundle branch (LBB), and then across to the right bundle branch (RBB), depolarising the intraventricular septum as it travels.

PURKINJE FIBRES

The Purkinje fibres are specialised nerve cells that allow the impulse to pass through the ventricles, depolarising the mass of the ventricles.

MECHANISMS OF HEART FAILURE

The heart maintains blood pressure by two means, systemic vascular resistance and cardiac output. Cardiac output is controlled by stroke volume and heart rate. This can be summarised in two equations:

Blood pressure = systemic vascular resistance × cardiac output
Cardiac output = stroke volume × heart rate

Terminology

Systemic vascular resistance – The resistance that the left ventricle must overcome to pump blood around the systemic circulation.
Cardiac output – The amount of blood ejected from the ventricle in systole.
Stroke volume – The amount of blood pumped out by the ventricle in each contraction.
Contractility – Pumping action of the heart.

If cardiac output is compromised, compensatory mechanisms are activated. This can be life-saving in some situations, such as acute haemorrhage, but when heart disease is bad enough to compromise cardiac output, these mechanisms are constantly activated, and can cause CHF. There are two main systems that are triggered when cardiac output decreases, the neurohormonal system, also called the renin-angiotensin-aldosterone

Table 1.1 Actions of the compensatory mechanisms

Renin-angiotensin-aldosterone system	Adrenergic system
Vasoconstriction	Increase heart rate
Sodium retention	Increase contractility
Water retention	Vasoconstriction

system (RAAS), and the adrenergic system, also known as the sympathetic nervous system. A summary of the actions of the compensatory mechanisms can be seen in Table 1.1.

RAAS

When cardiac output is compromised, the juxtaglomerular apparatus of the kidney releases renin into the bloodstream. The production of renin causes angiotensinogen to form angiotensin I. The lungs convert angiotensin I to angiotensin II by the angiotensin-converting enzyme (ACE). Angiotensin II is now able to increase total peripheral resistance by vasoconstriction. Angiotensin II also acts at the hypothalamus, where it stimulates thirst. This makes the patient drink more, increasing fluid volume and therefore increasing blood pressure. Angiotensin II also increases the secretion of the anti-diuretic hormone (ADH), from the posterior pituitary gland. This concentrates urine, so less fluid is lost. Angiotensin II also stimulates the adrenergic, or sympathetic system, and sends messages to the adrenal cortex to stimulate the production of aldosterone. Table 1.2 summarises the effects of angiotensin II.

ROLE OF ALDOSTERONE

Aldosterone is a steroid hormone that acts on the collecting duct in the nephron of the kidney. It selectively retains sodium, thereby preventing its excretion, and water remains with sodium. In exchange for sodium retention, potassium is excreted in the urine. Therefore, increased aldosterone levels equals lower potassium in the blood, and extra fluid volume because of the increased water. This means that patients receiving diuresis because of heart failure can become hypokalaemic.

ADRENERGIC SYSTEM (ANS)

The adrenergic system, also known as the sympathetic nervous system, is also activated when blood pressure demands are not met. The ANS releases noradrenaline, which

Table 1.2 Summary of the effects of angiotensin II

- Vasoconstriction
- Acts at the hypothalamus, stimulating thirst
- Increases stimulation of ADH
- Stimulates adrenergic system
- Acts on the adrenal cortex to stimulate the release of aldosterone

makes the heart work harder by increasing heart rate, increasing contractility, and also increases vasoconstriction. In a healthy heart, the ANS can promptly restore cardiac output. However, if the heart is diseased, it is likely that chronic activation of the ANS will not meet metabolic demands because the heart has to continue working harder and harder in a vicious cycle to maintain sufficient output.

PRESENTATION OF PATIENTS WITH HEART FAILURE

CHF is said to be present when abnormal fluid has accumulated. Clinical signs will vary due to the amount of fluid, from patient to patient, and can also differ with species, but it is possible to see how compensatory mechanisms are activated, and the effect it has when patients present with heart failure. Further, because heart disease is often a slow progressive disease (excluding arrhythmias), patients can often adapt and seem to cope with abnormal fluid accumulation. When a patient is diagnosed with heart failure, it is almost impossible to reverse and needs to be managed with medication for the rest of the pet's life. If the patient is stable on medication, it is said that they are in compensated heart failure (Figure 1.7). If a patient is unstable, presenting in acute respiratory distress, it is said they are in decompensated heart failure, i.e., that the compensatory mechanisms are insufficient to maintain cardiac output (Figure 1.8).

Diseases that cause left-sided CHF are:

- Myxomatous mitral valve disease
- Dilated cardiomyopathy
- Hypertrophic cardiomyopathy
- Patent ductus arteriosus
- Aortic stenosis
- Mitral valve dysplasia

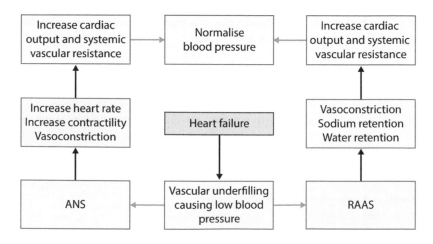

Figure 1.7 Cycle of compensated heart failure.

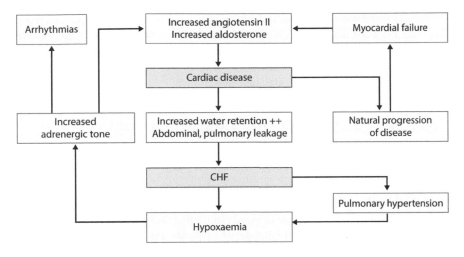

Figure 1.8 Cycle of decompensated heart failure.

Diseases that cause right-sided CHF are:

- Pulmonic stenosis
- Tricuspid valve disease or dysplasia

An important variation is how cats may present in heart failure. Due to a difference in their pulmonary vasculature, cats may present with pulmonary oedema, or pleural effusion as a result of left-sided CHF. This can mean that thoracocentesis may or may not be needed depending upon where the fluid has accumulated. The difference can easily be auscultated because with pulmonary oedema, crackles can be heard over lung fields, and pleural effusion presents with dull heart sounds on the ventral sternum. Table 1.3 summarises the clinical signs of left and right sided heart failure, and cats.

Table 1.3 Clinical signs associated with congestive heart failure

Left-sided heart failure – Pulmonary congestion	Right-sided heart failure – System venous congestion	Cats
Increased respiratory rate and effort	Increased respiratory rate and effort	Increased respiratory rate and effort
Tachypnoea	Tachypnoea	Tachypnoea
Respiratory distress	Dyspnoea	Respiratory distress
Pulmonary oedema	Ascites	Pulmonary oedema
Cough	Pleural and/or pericardial effusion	Pleural and/or pericardial effusion
Reduced exercise tolerance	Jugular distention	Depression or reduced activity
Syncope	Reduced exercise tolerance	Aortic thromboembolism
Anorexia	Syncope	Syncope
Weight and muscle loss		

In advanced disease, both dogs and cats can present with bilateral heart failure, resulting from left-sided disease. This is usually caused by substantially increased pressures in the left atrium that cause high pressure in the pulmonary artery, causing pulmonary hypertension. The increased pressure then backs up into the right ventricle and right atrium and into the systemic circulation.

CAUSES OF CONGESTIVE HEART FAILURE

CHF can occur from the following cardiac causes:

- *Systolic dysfunction* – Inability of the ventricles to contract effectively in systole. Seen with dilated cardiomyopathy when the ventricular myocardium becomes weak.
- *Volume overload* – An increase in blood volume that the ventricles must eject. Occurs with myxomatous mitral valve disease, when blood leaks back into the atrium in systole because the valves fail to close properly. Cardiac output is compromised, causing activation of the compensatory mechanisms to retain fluid. This causes an increase in circulating fluid volume.
- *Pressure overload* – An increase in pressure on the heart when the ventricles pump blood into the arteries. This can occur with stenosis of either the aortic or pulmonary arteries, or systemic or pulmonary hypertension.
- *Diastolic dysfunction* – Inability of the ventricles to relax and fill in diastole. Seen with hypertrophic cardiomyopathy when the ventricles become stiff and less compliant, or with pericardial effusion, when there is not enough space for the ventricles to fill.

FORWARD FAILURE

Occasionally, compensatory mechanisms do not get activated in time, such as may happen with an arrhythmia. If the heart rate is too fast or too slow, the heart may not have time to fill or be fast enough to meet blood pressure demands. This is known as forward or output failure. Sometimes, advanced cardiac disease may also cause forward failure. For example, chordae tendinea can rupture as a result of myxomatous mitral valve disease,

Table 1.4 Clinical signs associated with forward heart failure

Forward or output failure
Weakness
Collapse
Dyspnoea
Apnoea
Pallor
Irregular heart rhythm
Poor or absent pulse

or ventricles become non-compliant, as may be seen with hypertrophic cardiomyopathy or dilated cardiomyopathy. Patients with forward failure will often present collapsed. Chapter 8 considers emergency cardiac first aid. Table 1.4 summarises clinical signs seen with forward failure.

KEY POINTS

- The function of the heart is to provide oxygenated blood and nutrients to the body and meet blood pressure demands.
- The heart has four chambers and four heart valves. These work synchronously to maximise efficiency.
- Each chamber has a different intracardiac pressure, relating to its function.
- The conduction system initiates the heartbeat by an electrical impulse.
- Disease processes can cause compensatory mechanisms to occur. These mechanisms can lead to heart failure.
- Clinical signs vary from patient to patient and the severity of the disease. Clinical signs also differ depending upon where the disease process occurs. Left-sided CHF is the most common presentation in small animal medicine.

FURTHER READING

BSAVA Manual of Canine and Feline Cardiorespiratory Medicine, 2nd edition (2010). British Small Animal Veterinary Association, Gloucester.

(2)

Acquired heart disease in dogs

Acquired heart disease is the most common type of heart disease diagnosed in dogs. This chapter will focus on the two main diseases seen in dogs, myxomatous mitral valve disease (MMVD) and dilated cardiomyopathy (DCM). MMVD accounts for up to 70% of canine heart disease seen in general practice[1]. DCM is often a silent disease until clinical signs of heart failure occur, and then prognosis is poor. Both MMVD and DCM are diseases that most commonly affect the left side of the heart. As seen in Chapter 1, the left heart works with higher pressures to provide blood around the body, to maintain blood pressure. If the left heart is compromised, clinical signs of congestive left sided heart failure or forward failure can occur. Pericardial disease is also discussed in this chapter, as this can be a presentation nurses might experience.

MYXOMATOUS MITRAL VALVE DISEASE (MMVD)

Terminology

Different names have been used to describe the mitral valve in veterinary nursing textbooks. Often the tricuspid and mitral valves are discussed collectively and called the atrioventricular valves. Endocardiosis is a term used previously to describe degeneration of both the mitral and tricuspid valves but is not used today, because it is more accurate to assess the valves separately.

In an old paper[2], still cited by leading cardiologists, the breakdown of valvular degeneration was recorded as:

- Mitral valve alone – 62%
- Mitral and tricuspid valves – 32.5%
- Tricuspid valve alone – 1.3%

However, there are still many differences in terminology even when referring to one valve. Box 2.1 lists other names used to describe acquired disease. The American College of Veterinary Internal Medicine consensus statement (2019) uses the term MMVD[3], so this term shall be used here.

SIGNALMENT

The reason why MMVD occurs in some dogs is unknown. Affected dogs are born with normal mitral valve apparatus, but degenerative changes occur over time. It is a disease

DOI: 10.1201/9781003122173-3

BOX 2.1: Alternative names to describe mitral valve disease

NAMES FOR MMVD

Mitral valve disease
Degenerative mitral valve disease
Myxomatous mitral valve disease
Chronic mitral valve fibrosis
Chronic degenerative valvular disease*
Chronic valvular disease*
Endocardiosis*

*Names including both the mitral and tricuspid valves.

---

that mainly affects small to medium size breed dogs, but some larger breed dogs can also be affected. Breeds predisposed are shown in Box 2.2. A genetic link has been found in Cavalier King Charles Spaniels and Dachshunds, but as many as 85% of dogs over the age of 13 have MMVD[1]. Males seem to be predisposed to MMVD.

Aetiology

The mitral valve is located between the left atrium and left ventricle. The valve is a combination of structures known as the mitral valve apparatus. There are six components to the mitral valve apparatus, which work together to optimise left ventricular systolic function. Figure 2.1 shows a labelled mitral valve.

1. Posterior left atrial wall
2. Mitral annulus – The ring of tissue from which the mitral leaflets are suspended
3. Mitral valve leaflets
4. Chordae tendineae
5. Left ventricular papillary muscles
6. Left ventricular myocardium

Degeneration of the mitral valve apparatus occurs gradually over time, causing malformation of the apparatus and biomechanical dysfunction. As the apparatus degenerates, the mitral valve leaflets become unable to close properly. Therefore, when blood is

---

BOX 2.2: Breeds predisposed to MMVD

Cavalier King Charles Spaniel
Dachshund
Poodle
Chihuahua
Papillon
Whippet

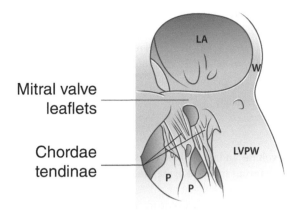

Mitral valve
leaflets

Chordae
tendinae

Figure 2.1 Diagram of labelled mitral valve. LA = Left atrium. W = Wall. LVPW = Left ventricular posterior wall. P = Papillary muscle.

ejected from the left ventricle into the aorta and around the body in systole, some blood flows back into the left atrium. This pattern of blood flow is called mitral regurgitation, and is the most common finding in MMVD. It is this regurgitant jet that causes the heart murmur sound. The greater the degenerative changes, the larger the volume of regurgitation, the louder the heart murmur. Figure 2.2 shows a mitral regurgitation jet on echocardiography. When the amount of blood leaving the ventricle decreases, cardiac output becomes compromised. This is when compensatory mechanisms are activated to increase

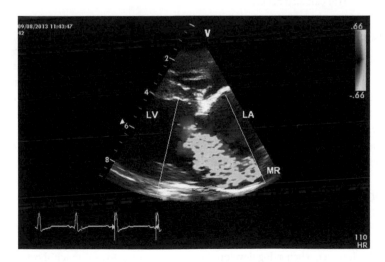

Figure 2.2 Mitral valve regurgitation seen on echocardiography. The large volume of green seen in the figure is the amount of blood flowing back into the left atrium in systole, instead of out through the aorta. LA = Left atrium. LV − Left ventricle. MR = Mitral regurgitation.

Table 2.1 Compensatory mechanisms activated in when cardiac output is compromised

Adrenergic system	Neurohormonal system or renin-angiotensin-aldosterone system
Increase heart rate	Vasoconstriction
Increase contractility	Sodium retention
Vasoconstriction	Water retention

circulating blood volume and meet blood pressure requirements. Table 2.1 describes the compensatory mechanisms involved in maximising cardiac output. Chapter 1 covers this process in more detail.

As the disease advances, volume overload of the left heart occurs, leading to remodelling of the left atria and left ventricle. As the left atrium and left ventricle dilate to accommodate the extra volume, the mitral valve apparatus is forced apart, increasing the volume of regurgitation. The greater the regurgitant jet, the more the compensatory mechanisms are activated to increase fluid volume. This is known as closed loop degeneration. In advanced disease, congestive heart failure and arrhythmias can occur, and chordae tendineae can rupture due to the additional stress. Forward, or output failure, can occur when there is insufficient cardiac output despite activation of the compensatory mechanisms.

Another complication that can occur as a result of left sided congestive heart failure (L-CHF) is pulmonary hypertension. This occurs partly because of the increased pressures in the left atrium, and also as a consequence of pulmonary arterial vasoconstriction reacting to hypoxia. This can exacerbate clinical signs of L-CHF, such as syncope, exercise intolerance, or dyspnoea. In advanced cases of MMVD, right sided congestive heart failure (R-CHF) can also occur.

CLINICAL SIGNS

MMVD is characterised by a left sided apical heart murmur, which gets louder as the disease progresses. A dog diagnosed with MMVD can be asymptomatic for many years, and may never succumb to the disease. If the disease does progress, exercise intolerance and lethargy can occur. Sometimes a cough is present, but this can also be an indicator of airway disease, which small dogs are predisposed to, so this needs to be excluded. If the disease progresses further, L-CHF and sometimes, R-CHF can occur. Box 2.3 summarises the clinical signs associated with MMVD.

PROGNOSIS

Many dogs can live for many years asymptomatically with MMVD. One study showed that dogs diagnosed with MMVD lived up to five and a half years[4] after a diagnosis of MMVD. However, when a dog develops heart failure, prognosis is much shorter. Despite advances in pre-clinical heart failure treatment, survival times from onset of heart failure signs is 6–14 months.[5] MMVD is unpredictable in its progression, and therefore not all dogs with MMVD will deteriorate.

> **BOX 2.3: Clinical signs of heart failure resulting from MMVD**
>
> - *Heart murmur* – usually grade IV – VI/VI when heart failure present
> - Cough
> - Tachypnoea, respiratory distress, orthopnoea
> - Lethargy
> - Anorexia
> - Reduced exercise tolerance
> - Syncope
> - *Weight and muscle loss* – At advanced stages of the disease
> - *Arrhythmias* – Most commonly ventricular premature complexes and atrial fibrillation
> - *Ascites* – If R-CHF develops (an example is shown in Figure 2.3)
> - Forward failure signs in extreme cases – weakness, collapse, pallor, poor or absent pulse

NURSING AND TREATMENT OF MMVD

The American College of Veterinary Internal Medicine consensus statement (2019)[2] categorised MMVD in to four separate stages. This is helpful because it outlines treatment and nursing guidelines that can be adapted into everyday practice. Table 2.2 summarises the different stages described in the consensus statement.

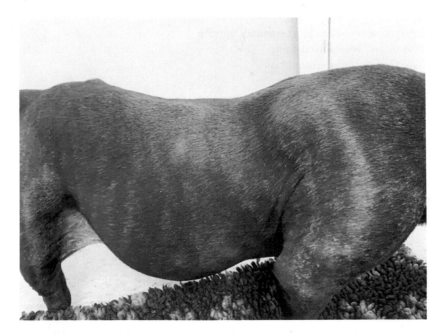

Figure 2.3 Picture of dog with ascites. Note the distended abdomen.

Table 2.2 Classification of MMVD

Stage	Classification criteria	Description
A	At risk	Dogs at high risk of developing MMVD due to their breed but have no evidence of heart disease.
B	Heart disease present, but no heart failure	Two distinct categories in this stage: B1 – Audible heart murmur on auscultation, but no echocardiographic or radiographic changes. B2 – Audible heart murmur on auscultation, but echocardiographic and/or radiographic changes associated with mitral valve disease present, such as left sided enlargement.
C	Heart failure	Either past or current heart failure. A wide group ranging from the dog managed on medication and treated as an outpatient, to the patient in acute, life-threatening heart failure.
D	Refractory heart failure	Routine heart failure medication no longer effective.

RECOMMENDATIONS OF NURSING AND TREATMENT OF STAGE A DOGS

Stage A dogs are those at high risk of developing MMVD due to their breed. Figure 2.4 shows a heart on echocardiography with no mitral valve degeneration. Guidelines include:-

- Annual auscultation by a veterinary surgeon
- No dietary recommendations
- No treatment recommendations

RECOMMENDATIONS OF NURSING AND TREATMENT OF STAGE B DOGS

Dogs in stage B have structural heart disease, but crucially, do not have clinical signs of heart failure. This class has been subdivided into two sections, B1 and B2. Figure 2.5 shows B2 on echocardiography, where the mitral valve is thickened, and the left atrium and ventricle are dilated.

B1 – DOGS WITH A MURMUR BUT NO CARDIAC CHANGES NOTED ON ECHOCARDIOGRAPHY OR RADIOGRAPHY

Diagnostic tests

- Thoracic radiography is recommended to obtain a baseline for the individual patient. This can also highlight if airway disease is present.
- Blood pressure measurement to establish a baseline and rule out concurrent hypertension.
- Echocardiography to conclusively diagnose the cause of the murmur, and measure chamber size, and assess regurgitant flow through the mitral valve.

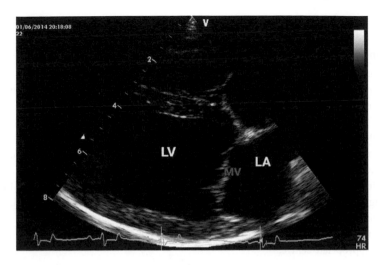

Figure 2.4 Echocardiographic image of a normal canine heart. Note the size of the left ventricle (LV) and left atrium (LA), and how the mitral valve (MV) is thin, closes fully and does not protrude into the left atrium. The left atrium should fit approximately twice in the space of the left ventricle.

Nursing and treatment recommendations

- No dietary recommendations
- No treatment recommendations
- Assessment every 6–12 months to assess progression of disease

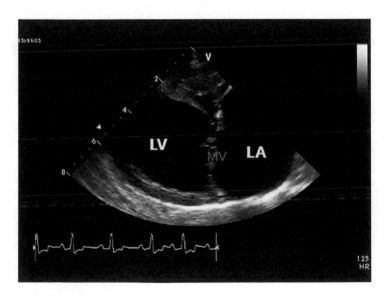

Figure 2.5 Echocardiographic image of MMVD at stage B2. Note the increased size of the left atrium (LA) and left ventricle (LV), and the mitral valve (MV) is visibly thickened.

B2 – DOGS WITH A MURMUR AND HAVE CARDIAC CHANGES ON ECHOCARDIOGRAPHY OR RADIOGRAPHY

Diagnostic tests

- A murmur equal to or greater than III/VI
- Echocardiographic confirmation of left atrial and/or left ventricular enlargement
- Vertebral heart score greater than 10.5 (using breed appropriate scoring)

Nursing and treatment recommendations

- Pimobendan every 12 hours. Pimobendan is a positive inotrope that increases contractility and helps the ventricle pump more effectively.
- Dietary change is recommended. Diet should moderately restrict sodium, be highly palatable, and contain adequate protein and calories to maximise body condition.
- If mitral valve surgery is an option to the owner, this is where referral can be made to an appropriate centre.

RECOMMENDATIONS OF NURSING AND TREATMENT OF STAGE C DOGS

This stage is reached when the dog has, or has had, clinical signs of CHF due to MMVD. This group includes dogs with chronic heart failure that are being managed on heart failure medication, and those in acute life-threatening heart failure. The nursing management of these patients varies on presentation. Figure 2.6 shows left atrial (LA) and ventricular (LV) dilation, with a stretched and thickened mitral valve (MV).

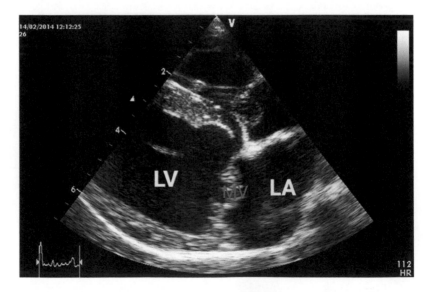

Figure 2.6 Echocardiographic image of MMVD at stage C. Note that the left atrium (LA) and left ventricle (LV) are dilated, and the mitral valve (MV) is stretched and bowing into the left atrium.

DIAGNOSTIC TESTS

- Radiographs to rule out concurrent tracheobronchial disease.
- Baseline laboratory tests, to include total protein and packed cell volume, creatinine, urea nitrogen, electrolytes, and urine specific gravity.
- Echocardiography can be used to confirm MMVD, measure chamber sizes, assess contractility, and assess if pulmonary hypertension present.
- Blood pressure to assess cardiac output.
- Serum NT-proBNP can be measured if diagnosis of MMVD is unsure. High concentrations would indicate heart disease, low concentrations respiratory disease.

ACUTE AND LIFE-THREATENING HEART FAILURE – NURSING AND TREATMENT RECOMMENDATIONS

Cardiac emergencies are covered in more detail in Chapter 8.

- Oxygen supplementation, in as stress-free manner as possible.
- Furosemide (2 mg/kg) to be administered either intravenously (IV), if access can be gained without stressing the patient, or intramuscularly (IM) until IV access can be achieved. Furosemide can be given hourly until respiratory rate improves, or until a total dose of 8 mg/kg has been given over four hours. Furosemide can be given as boluses or as a continuous rate infusion (CRI).
- Access to plentiful water and checked regularly for urination. If changing bedding, stress should be minimised.
- Pimobendan (0.25–0.3 mg/kg q12) should be started if the patient is not already on it. Outside of the United States, an IV preparation is available.
- Sedation may be necessary if patient is distressed. Butorphanol (0.2–0.25 mg/kg) IV or IM is most commonly recommended.
- Optimal nursing care, including monitoring the environmental temperature if using an oxygen chamber, changing bedding, raising the head on bedding, and resting in sternal recumbency if sedated.
- Dobutamine (2.5–10 µg/kg/min as a CRI, starting at 2.5 µg/kg/minute, increasing the dosage incrementally) might be indicated if the patient does not respond to the measures listed above. If used, continuous electrocardiography (ECG) should be attached and monitored. Dobutamine can have pro-arrhythmic effects and should be reduced and removed if this occurs.
- Sodium nitroprusside as a CRI (1–15 µg/kg/minute) may also be prescribed, if life threatening pulmonary oedema is not resolving. This also requires constant ECG and blood pressure monitoring.

CHRONIC HEART FAILURE – NURSING AND TREATMENT RECOMMENDATIONS

- Administer per os medication – furosemide, pimobendan, and others if prescribed, such as an angiotensin converting enzyme inhibitors to block neurohormonal activation, or sildenafil, to reduce pulmonary hypertension.
- Regular measurement of serum creatinine, urea nitrogen, and electrolytes.
- Initiate a home care plan with the owner to promote appetite, optimise ideal body weight, monitor sleeping respiratory rate, and clear instructions on what medication

is to be given and when, including when it might need adjustment, such as if the sleeping respiratory rate increases.

- Arrhythmia management and/or assessment by 24-hour ECG may be indicated.

DIETARY RECOMMENDATIONS

Patients often become inappetent when heart failure is present, and cardiac cachexia can occur. Cardiac cachexia is defined as muscle or lean body mass loss due to heart failure, and has been shown to be a negative prognostic indicator[2]. It is recommended to try and avoid cardiac cachexia from developing in the first instance. Figure 2.7 shows an example of cachexia in a dog with MMVD. The consensus statement suggests:

- Maintain calorie intake, recommended at 60 kcal/kg. To encourage inappetent dogs to eat, methods such as warming food, offering a variety of food types and mixing wet and dry food.
- Use adequate protein diets, avoiding low protein ones, unless renal failure is also present.
- Other causes of inappetence should be ruled out, such as drug induced causes or concurrent disease.
- Record and monitor body weight, body condition score and muscle condition score on each visit.
- Modest sodium restriction. When discussing the diet plan with owners, all treats or table scraps that might be used to administer medication should be included.

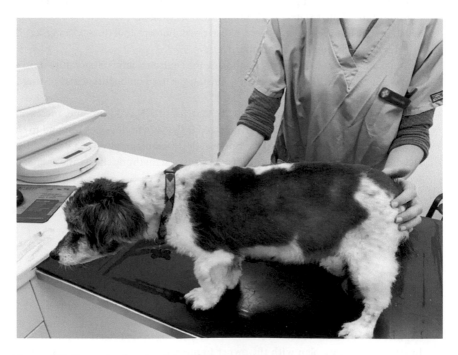

Figure 2.7 Example of cachexia in a dog.

RECOMMENDATIONS OF NURSING AND TREATMENT OF STAGE D DOGS

Patients that are classified at stage D are not responding to standard heart failure medication any longer. As with stage C patients, class D patients can also present in acute, life-threatening heart failure or chronic heart failure.

DIAGNOSTIC TESTS

Same as class C patients.

ACUTE AND LIFE THREATENING REFRACTORY HEART FAILURE – NURSING AND TREATMENT RECOMMENDATIONS

Very similar to class C acute heart failure patients, in that stress must be avoided and oxygen supplementation may be necessary. Due to increased drug doses attempting to control clinical signs, increased monitoring may be necessary to observe renal and electrolyte parameters. With increased urination, potassium loss may increase, resulting in hypokalaemia. Cavity centesis may be necessary to remove effusions to make the patient more comfortable. If arterial dilators are used, such as dobutamine, blood pressure needs to be closely monitored to avoid hypotension. Systolic blood pressure should remain over 85 mmHg, mean arterial pressure over 60 mmHg.

CHRONIC REFRACTORY HEART FAILURE – NURSING AND TREATMENT RECOMMENDATIONS

Dogs with chronic refractory heart failure will require regular monitoring to assess for potential side effects of the various medications they may be prescribed, such as renal and electrolyte parameters and blood pressure. Weight and body and muscle condition scores should also be recorded.

DIETARY RECOMMENDATIONS

As for stage C, but for those with refractory effusions, further sodium restriction is recommended, if this does not compromise appetite.

The nurse's role at stage D is to promote quality of life, and support the owner.

DILATED CARDIOMYOPATHY (DCM)

The underlying cause of DCM is unknown, and so diagnosis is often made after ruling out other possible causes. Other causes of DCM, known as secondary cardiomyopathies, include toxins, the chemotherapy drug doxorubicin, nutritional deficiencies such as taurine, some systemic diseases such as hypothyroidism, and infectious diseases like Bartonella. These causes need to be ruled out before a diagnosis of primary DCM can be given, because this can affect treatment options.

Table 2.3 Breeds with a high prevalence of DCM

Giant breeds	Large breeds	Spaniel breeds	Other
Irish Wolfhound	Doberman	English Cocker Spaniel	Portuguese
Deerhound	Boxer	English Springer Spaniel	Water Dog
Great Dane	Weimaraner	American Cocker Spaniel	
Newfoundland	Dogue de Bordeaux		
St Bernard	Golden Retriever		
Leonberger	Labrador Retriever		
	Old English Sheepdog		
	German Shepherd Dog		

SIGNALMENT

DCM is an inherited disease, and there does seem to be some breed predisposition. It is most commonly diagnosed in medium-large breed dogs, but English and American Cocker Spaniels can also be affected. Table 2.3 lists breeds with a high prevalence of DCM. It has recently been reported in America that there may be a link between dogs being fed boutique, exotic and/or grain free diets and DCM[6]. There is no clear link between diet and DCM at present, but DCM has been reported in atypical breeds.

There does not appear to be a sex predisposition to DCM, but males are more likely to present with congestive heart failure at a younger age. The average age of diagnosis is between four and eight years old, but some dogs can be younger.

AETIOLOGY

Cardiomyopathy is a term applied to any cardiac disorder caused by myocardial dysfunction. DCM is an acquired myocardial disease, characterised by ventricular dilation and poor systolic function, often starting in the left ventricle. DCM affects the heart's ability to pump blood around the body because the myocardium is unable to contract properly. This myocardial weakness can lead to a decrease in cardiac output because the ventricle is unable to push blood through the aorta at the pressure required. As with MMVD, as soon as blood pressure requirements are not met, the body activates compensatory mechanisms. These mechanisms increase heart rate, retain fluid and improve the heart's contractility, by making the ventricles pump harder. This can result in ventricular dilation, often distorting the mitral valve apparatus, and allowing a regurgitant jet of blood to flow back into the left atrium each time the heart pumps in systole. The more the atria and ventricles become dilated, the larger the regurgitation jet becomes, the more compensatory mechanisms are triggered. Just as with MMVD, the extra fluid can cause pressure overload in the lungs, resulting in pulmonary oedema, and other clinical signs of L-CHF, and can also sometimes cause high right sided pressures, leading to pulmonary hypertension and R-CHF.

Ventricular arrhythmias are also a common finding with DCM, and sudden death can occur as a result. Ventricular premature complexes are often observed, as well as more complex ventricular rhythms, such as couplets, triplets, ventricular runs, or ventricular

Table 2.4 Stages of DCM

Stages of DCM	Clinical findings
At risk	Dogs that are at risk of developing DCM due to their breed, but have no evidence of DCM on echocardiography, and no abnormalities on electrocardiography (ECG). Dogs do not have any clinical signs of heart disease.
Occult or 'pre-clinical'	Ventricular premature complexes are seen on ECG. And/or Echocardiographic change, such as left ventricular dilatation. Dogs do not have any clinical signs of heart disease.
Overt	Clinical signs of heart failure, and/or arrhythmias.

tachycardia. It has been shown that Dobermans are at particular risk of ventricular arrhythmias, and this has been linked to the higher mortality rate in this breed[7]. Atrial fibrillation may also occur in advanced disease, when the atrial myocardium has been stretched.

STAGING OF DCM

DCM is described as having distinct stages. Table 2.4 summarises these stages.

CLINICAL SIGNS

Clinical signs can vary from asymptomatic to heart failure or sudden death. The occult stage of the disease can progress slowly, where the only evidence of DCM is on echocardiography

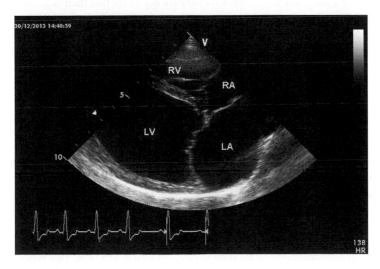

Figure 2.8 DCM seen on echocardiography. Note the enlargement of the left atrium and ventricle, the thin left ventricular wall and how stretched the mitral valve is in this image.

BOX 2.4: Clinical signs of DCM

- Tachypnoea, respiratory distress, orthopnoea
- Cough – sometimes producing pink froth
- Exercise intolerance
- Syncope
- Collapse
- Left apical systolic heart murmur
- Arrhythmias such as atrial fibrillation or ventricular rhythms
- Poor appetite
- Weight and muscle loss – at advanced stages of the disease
- Ascites or pleural effusion if R-CHF occurs
- Sudden death

---

or ECG. The classic heart murmur auscultated with MMVD is not as helpful with DCM. This is because the heart murmur sound is related to the amount of blood flowing across the mitral valve (mitral regurgitation) back into the left atrium during systole, when it should be ejected out through the aorta. By the time a heart murmur can be heard in a DCM patient, the heart has undergone significant remodelling, effectively pulling the mitral valve apart because of the dilation. Figure 2.8 shows DCM on echocardiography, where left sided dilation are present. However, like MMVD, DCM primarily affects the left side of the heart, so there are many similarities in the clinical signs. Box 2.4 shows those commonly seen.

Prognosis

DCM can be a silent disease, so often owners are not aware that their dog has heart disease, until it develops heart failure, collapses or even dies suddenly. As the heart murmur may not develop until severe cardiac remodelling has occurred, it often means that DCM is not diagnosed until advanced disease is present. Survival times for dogs diagnosed with congestive heart failure resulting from DCM is 2–4 months[8]. For dogs predisposed to DCM, screening programmes are available.

Diagnostic tests

The European Society of Veterinary Cardiology has developed guidelines for Dobermans[9], but these can be extrapolated to all breeds predisposed to DCM. It has been recognised that echocardiography is a difficult and costly diagnostic test, and so may not be possible for all patients. Alternative diagnostic tests have been suggested.

Recommended diagnostic tests

- Annual echocardiography for dogs at risk, aged three and over. This is because one-off screening cannot rule out future development of DCM. Echocardiography can be used to record baseline cardiac parameters and chart progression of the disease.

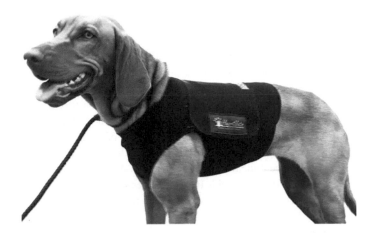

Figure 2.9 Dog wearing a 24-hour Holter ECG monitor.

Echocardiography can measure chamber size, ventricular function, valve function, and mitral regurgitation.

• 24-hour Holter ECG recording that is worn by the patient (Figure 2.9). This can identify the number, frequency and complexity of arrhythmias. Annual screening is recommended.

If echocardiography and Holter monitoring are unavailable, then other diagnostic tests may be useful, such as blood sampling for the cardiac biomarkers, N-Terminal pro B-type natriuretic peptide (NTproBNP) and cardiac troponin I (cTnI). NTproBNP is released in response to atrial and ventricular myocardial stretch, and cardiac troponins are a protein found when myocardial cells have been damaged or have died. In the case of both tests, the higher the number, the higher the risk of heart disease.

RECOMMENDATIONS OF NURSING AND TREATMENT OF DCM

Screening is recommended so that only healthy dogs are bred from. One report showed that 58.8% of Dobermans in Europe were affected by DCM, so client education is crucial[6]. Whilst annual screening may be cost prohibitive for some clients, they should be made aware of such programmes. Another reason for at risk breeds to be screened is that pimobendan can be prescribed at the occult stage, which has been shown to increase survival time. When a patient reaches heart failure, the same nursing and treatment used in stage C and D of MMVD can be applied. However, the increased risk of arrhythmias should be noted, making it even more important to reduce stress and exercise. Due to the often later diagnosis of DCM when advanced disease is present, and the poor prognosis after diagnosis, clients may need additional support.

PERICARDIAL DISEASE

Pericardial effusions can be seen in veterinary practice. In dogs, pericardial effusion can be due to rare types of congenital disease, such as peritoneal-pericardial-diaphragmatic hernia (PPDH). Acquired disease is more common however, and the most frequent cause is neoplasia, either haemangiosarcoma of the right atrium or chemodectoma affecting the heart base. Idiopathic disease is the second most common cause of pericardial effusion in dogs. In cats, pericardial effusion is most commonly diagnosed as a result of congestive heart failure.

Depending upon the amount of fluid present within the pericardium, or occlusion by a mass, the heart can have difficulty filling in diastole. As intracardiac pressures in the right atrium are the lowest, it is possible in severe cases sometimes, to see the right atrial free wall collapse on echocardiography. This is called cardiac tamponade.

CLINICAL SIGNS

Patients can present with vague signs of lethargy to collapse. Other signs include inappetence, weight loss, and respiratory difficulty.

DIAGNOSIS

Echocardiography is the best method for diagnosis. The hyperechoic fluid contrasts well against the heart structures. When fluid is present, it is also easier to detect lesions such as tumours. Radiography may show a spherical shaped heart that is football shaped. Electrocardiography may show 'electrical alternans', a sinus rhythm with alternating size QRS complexes, seen because of the heart swinging in the pericardial fluid.

NURSING AND TREATMENT RECOMMENDATIONS

Treatment depends upon diagnosis. Pericardiocentesis can be both therapeutic and provide diagnostic information. Chapter 8 covers emergency first aid, if pericardiocentesis is required.

KEY POINTS

- MMVD is the most common acquired heart disease seen in small animal practice.
- Dogs can live with MMVD asymptomatically for years, before if ever, progressing to heart failure.
- There are four stages of MMVD, all with nursing and treatment recommendations.
- DCM has been classified as having three stages. Screening and client education is important as the disease can be silent.
- Emergency cardiac nursing is covered in Chapter 8.

FURTHER READING

Keene BW, Atkins CE, Bonagura JD, Fox PR, Häggström J, Fuentes VL, Oyama MA, Rush JE, Stepien R, Uechi M (2019). ACVIM consensus guidelines for the diagnosis and treatment of myxomatous mitral valve disease in dogs. *Journal of Veterinary Internal Medicine.* May-Jun 33(3): 1113–1560.

Wess G, Domenech J, Dukes-McEwan J, Häggström J, Gordon S (2017). European Society of Veterinary Cardiology screening guidelines for dilated cardiomyopathy in Doberman Pinschers. *Journal of Veterinary Cardiology.* 19, 405–415.

REFERENCES

1. Häggström J (2010). Myxomatous mitral valve disease. In: Fuentes LV, Johnson LR, Dennis S, eds. *BSAVA Manual of Canine and Feline Cardiorespiratory Medicine,* 2nd edition. British Small Animal Veterinary Association, Gloucester: 186–194.
2. Buchanan JW (1977). Chronic valvular disease (endocardiosis) in dogs. *Advances in Veterinary Science and Comparative Medicine.* 21: 75–106.
3. Keene BW, Atkins CE, Bonagura JD, Fox PR, Häggström J, Fuentes VL, Oyama MA, Rush JE, Stepien R, Uechi M (2019). ACVIM consensus guidelines for the diagnosis and treatment of myxomatous mitral valve disease in dogs. *Journal of Veterinary Internal Medicine.* May-Jun 33(3): 1113–1560.
4. Borgarelli M, Crosara S, Lamb K, Savarino P, La Rosa G, Tarducci A, Häggström J (2012). Survival characteristics and prognostic variables of dogs with preclinical chronic degenerative mitral valve disease attributable to myxomatous degeneration. *Journal of Veterinary Internal Medicine.* Jan-Feb; 26(1): 69–75.
5. Beaumier A, Rush JE, Yang VK, Freeman LM (2018). Clinical findings and survival time in dogs with advanced heart failure. *Journal of Veterinary Internal Medicine.* May-Jun; 32(3): 944–950.
6. Adin D, DeFrancesco TC, Keene B, Tou S, Meurs K, Atkins C, Aona B, Kurtz K, Barron L, Saker K (2019). Echocardiographic phenotype of canine dilated cardiomyopathy differs based on diet type. *Journal of Veterinary Cardiology.* 21: 1–9.
7. Calvert CA, Jacobs GJ, Smith DD, Rathbun SL, Pickus CW (2000). Association between results of ambulatory electrocardiography and development of cardiomyopathy during long-term follow-up of Doberman pinschers. *Journal of the American Veterinary Medical Association.* 216(1): 34–39.
8. Martin MW, Stafford Johnson M, Strehlau G and King JN (2010). Canine dilated cardiomyopathy: a retrospective study of prognostic findings in 367 clinical cases. *Journal of Small Animal Practice.* Aug; 51 (8): 428–436.
9. Wess G, Domenech J, Dukes-McEwan J, Häggström J, Gordon S (2017). European Society of Veterinary Cardiology screening guidelines for dilated cardiomyopathy in Doberman Pinschers. *Journal of Veterinary Cardiology.* 19, 405–415.

3

Acquired heart disease in cats

Acquired heart disease is the most common type of heart disease diagnosed in cats. The American College of Veterinary Internal Medicine consensus statement (2020) standardised terminology and provided guidance on diagnosis for veterinary surgeons, but also provided easy to use nursing guidelines. The most common type of feline cardiomyopathy is hypertrophic cardiomyopathy (HCM).

TERMINOLOGY

Cardiomyopathy is a term applied to any cardiac disorder caused by myocardial dysfunction, but it is a broad term including different myocardial diseases, which have different phenotypes and prognosis. A phenotype is an observable and therefore measurable trait. By using the term phenotype, a veterinary surgeon can record the heart's appearance, but not presume the cause of these changes. For example, the heart can have a thick left ventricle and look like HCM, but the cause does not have to be HCM. This is relevant because there can be other causes of left ventricular hypertrophy, such as hyperthyroidism, hypertension, acromegaly or aortic stenosis. It is important to rule out other causes of hypertrophy, because treatment will vary.

There are other phenotypes reported in feline cardiology, such as dilated cardiomyopathy, restrictive cardiomyopathy, arrhythmogenic cardiomyopathy, but the HCM phenotype appears to predominate. However, the prevalence of the other phenotypes is not known. An explanation of the phenotypic groups is shown in Table 3.1. Phenotypic groups can change over time due to disease progression or the development of concurrent disease.

SIGNALMENT

HCM is the most common phenotype found in cats, and it is believed that there is a genetic link. Such a link has been found in Maine Coon and Ragdoll breeds. Breed predisposition can be found in Box 3.1.

HCM can be present at any age, but is more common in the middle aged to older cat. One study reported that the prevalence of HCM in the general cat population to be[2]:

- 6–12 months = 4.3%
- 1–3 years = 9.9%
- 3–9 years = 18.6%
- 9 years plus = 29.4%

This means that in this study, nearly one third of cats over the age of nine have HCM.

DOI: 10.1201/9781003122173-4

Table 3.1 Description of phenotypic groups in feline cardiology. These descriptions are based on echocardiographic findings[1]

Phenotype	Definition
Hypertrophic cardiomyopathy (HCM)	Diffuse or regional increased left ventricular wall thickness.
Restrictive cardiomyopathy (RCM)	Normal left ventricular measurements with left atrial or biatrial enlargement.
Dilated cardiomyopathy (DCM)	Left ventricular systolic dysfunction. Normal or dilated left ventricular wall thickness and atrial dilatation.
Arrhythmogenic cardiomyopathy (ARVC)	Severe right atrial and right ventricular dilatation. Arrhythmias and right sided congestive heart failure common.
Nonspecific phenotype	A cardiomyopathic phenotype that is not satisfactorily explained by the other groups.

AETIOLOGY

HCM is the most common phenotype reported in cats, and it is characterised by a thickened, or hypertrophied, left ventricle. When the ventricle becomes thickened, it becomes stiff and cannot relax as it should. If it cannot relax properly, it cannot fill with blood as it needs to in diastole. This underfilling can compromise cardiac output, activating compensatory mechanisms, to make the heart work harder and retain fluid to increase circulating volume. This creates extra pressure on the left side of the heart, stretching the left atrial muscle to accommodate the extra volume. This fluid can also cause congestion either in the lungs, causing pulmonary oedema, or in the pleural cavity, causing pleural effusion. This is when left sided congestive heart failure (L-CHF) occurs. In severe disease, congestion can back up from the lungs to the right side of the heart, causing systemic venous congestion, which may present as ascites, jugular distention or pericardial effusion.

Another consideration is that the thickness of the hypertrophied ventricle may exceed the local blood supply, and cause localised ischemia. This can increase the stiffness and inefficiency of the ventricle and cause arrhythmias. The pattern of hypertrophy can vary greatly in cats, ranging from localised areas of thickness, often on just the septal wall,

BOX 3.1: Breeds predisposed to HCM

Maine Coon
Ragdoll
Bengal
British Short Hair
Sphynx
Norwegian Forest

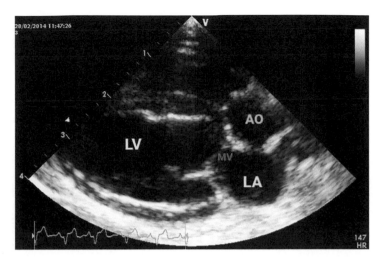

Figure 3.1 Normal cat heart on echocardiography, in right parasternal axis view. The left atrium (LA) is small and should be able to fit in to the left ventricle (LV) approximately twice. The ventricle has a cigar shape appearance. Ao = Aorta. MV = Mitral valve.

which is usually well tolerated, or to a more generalised hypertrophy affecting the whole ventricle. Examples of a normal cat heart on echocardiography compared to a HCM heart are seen in Figures 3.1–3.5.

A devasting consequence of left ventricular hypertrophy and atrial enlargement can be the development of a thrombus. As fluid volume increases the size of the left atrium,

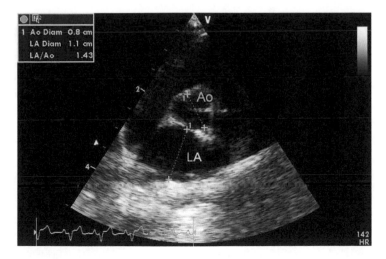

Figure 3.2 Normal cat heart on echocardiography in a different view (short axis), showing the left atrium (LA) to aorta (Ao) ratio. The aorta is in the middle of the picture, the left atrium is below. As an approximate, the left atrium should be the same size as the aorta, or up to one and a half times larger.

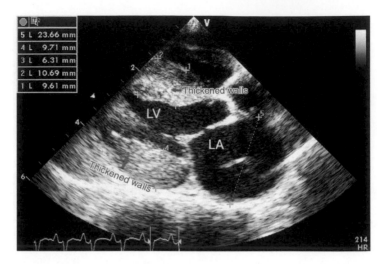

Figure 3.3 HCM on echocardiography, in right parasternal axis view. The left atrium (LA) is large and the ventricles are very thick.

blood slows down, unable to pass through the mitral valve and into the ventricle as quickly as it should. This slow-moving blood is called spontaneous echo contrast, and given its appearance on echocardiography, is often referred to as 'smoke' (Figure 3.5). The atrium has a teardrop-like structure, called the left atrial appendage. It is here that blood flow can slow down to a point of stopping. If this happens, a clot or thrombus forms (Figure 3.6). Parts of the thrombus can then dislodge and enter the systemic circulation,

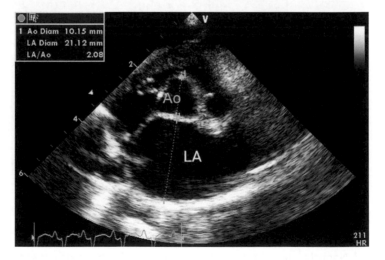

Figure 3.4 HCM on echocardiography showing the left atrium (LA) to aorta ratio (Ao) in short axis. The aorta is in the middle of the picture, the left atrium is below. The left atrium is considerably larger than the aorta.

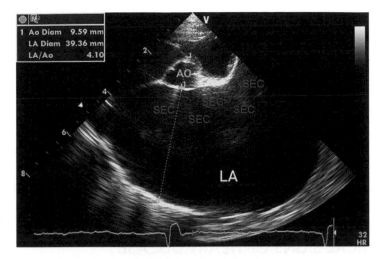

Figure 3.5 Echocardiographic picture of extremely large left atrium (LA) compared to the aorta (AO). The grey area under the aorta and to the right is spontaneous echo contrast (SEC).

ending up in the brain, mesentery, kidneys, brachial artery or the distal aorta. It can cause paresis or paralysis of forelimbs or hindlimbs, sometimes in one limb, sometimes both. Table 3.2 shows the results of a study recording the presentation of 250 cats diagnosed with a thrombus[3]. When the thrombus terminates in the distal aorta, it is known as an aortic thromboembolism (ATE), or saddle thrombus.

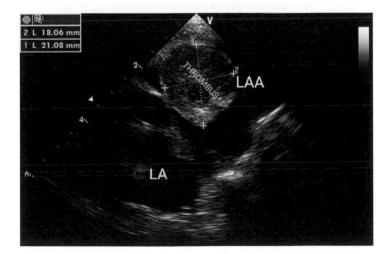

Figure 3.6 Echocardiographic picture of thrombus in left atrium (LA). This has occurred as a result of significant left atrial enlargement and lack of blood movement. LAA = left atrial appendage. LA = left atrium.

Table 3.2 Results of one study of 250 cats assessing limbs affected by aortic thromboembolism[3]

Limbs affected by ATE	Percent of cats affected %
Only right hind (RH)	6
Only left hind (LH)	6
RH and LH	77.6
Only right fore (RF)	4.8
Only left fore (LF)	4
RH, LH, and LF	0.8
RH, LH, RF, and LF	0.4
Missing data	0.4

CLINICAL SIGNS OF HEART DISEASE

Feline heart disease is often silent, and the first time an owner will know that their cat has heart disease is when it presents either dyspnoeic due to heart failure, vocalising loudly in distress with an ATE, or when it dies suddenly. Other clinical signs include depression or reduced activity (which often goes unnoticed as the cat may be aging), or syncope. Table 3.3 summarises the clinical signs present in feline heart disease. Table 3.4 the clinical signs associated with a thrombotic event. Figure 3.7 shows a cat with an ATE affecting the right hind limb

Table 3.3 Clinical signs of feline heart disease

No historical signs before presentation
Depression or reduced activity
Aortic thromboembolism
Congestive heart failure – respiratory distress due
  to pulmonary oedema or pleural effusion
Syncope
Sudden death

Table 3.4 Clinical signs of a thrombotic event

No historical signs prior to the episode
Acute onset of pain due to paralysis or paresis
Loss of peripheral pulses in affected limb(s)
Tissue pallor
Cold extremities of affected limb(s)
Signs of heart failure – including respiratory
  distress or tachypnoea
Hypothermia

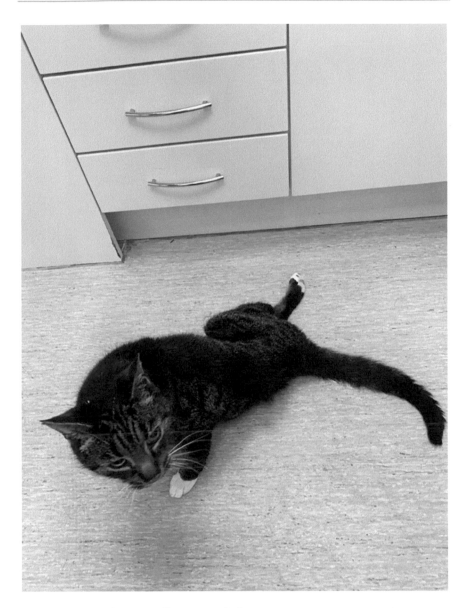

Figure 3.7 Cat with an ATE affecting one limb.

FINDINGS ON AUSCULTATION

A heart murmur is not a reliable indicator of heart disease because cats can have heart disease present, but have no murmur. A murmur is caused either by an obstruction to blood flow in the left ventricular outflow tract, such as an area of localised hypertrophy, or by the posterior mitral valve leaflet being sucked back into the left ventricular outflow

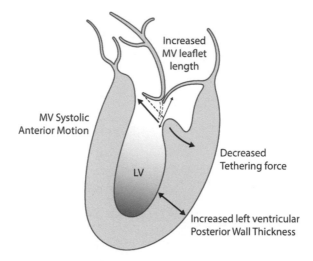

Figure 3.8 Diagram of SAM. When the mitral valve leaflet is sucked back into the left ventricular outflow tract, the origin of the aorta, this can cause a heart murmur. However, a localised area of hypertrophy in the same place would also cause an obstruction to blood flow and cause a heart murmur.

tract in systole. Hypertrophy in cats can be generalised or diffuse, and so may not necessarily cause an obstruction to blood flow, thus no murmur is heard. However, if the posterior mitral valve leaflet is sucked back into the left ventricular outflow tract, it will cause an audible murmur (Figure 3.8). This is called systolic anterior motion (SAM), and the loudness of the murmur is often related to heart rate. The faster the heart rate, the more the leaflet is drawn back into the outflow tract, and the louder the murmur. If the heart rate is slower, there is less force to pull the leaflet into the outflow tract. This will decrease the heart murmur sound, and it may even disappear altogether. SAM can occur without heart disease being present, therefore the cat may have a heart murmur, but no disease. It is not known exactly why SAM occurs, but one theory is that the posterior mitral valve leaflet is longer, so it gets sucked back under the high pressure of increased heart rates. Table 3.5 shows the correlation of heart disease and murmurs in healthy cats[4].

Audible arrhythmias may be heard and can be indicative of heart disease. An audible arrhythmia may sound like a missed beat (a ventricular premature complex), or like a

Table 3.5 Findings of a study investigating the prevalence of heart murmurs and heart disease in healthy cats[4]. Heart murmur prevalence in 199 healthy cats

Those with no heart disease present

- 34% had a heart murmur
- 66% had no heart murmur

Those with heart disease present

- 16% of cats had no heart murmur

fast irregular sound (atrial fibrillation). A gallop sound may be auscultated, and can be linked to heart disease. A gallop sound is an extra heart sound to the normal 'lub dub', and occurs when the atria contracts and blood hits a stiff ventricle wall. Gallop sounds can also be heard in older cats or those diagnosed with hyperthyroidism.

NURSING AND TREATMENT OF FELINE HEART DISEASE

The American College of Veterinary Internal Medicine published a consensus statement helping to guide classification, diagnosis and management of feline cardiomyopathies[1]. It outlines treatment and nursing guidelines that can be adapted into everyday practice. It also classified feline heart disease into categories (Table 3.6).

RECOMMENDATIONS OF NURSING AND TREATMENT OF STAGE A CATS

Stage A cats are those at risk of developing HCM due to their breed or family history.

- It is suggested that queens of high-risk breeds are assessed regularly by a cardiologist.
- Genetic tests performed where applicable.
- No treatment recommendations.

RECOMMENDATIONS OF NURSING AND TREATMENT OF STAGE B CATS

Stage B cats have increased left ventricular thickness, but no clinical signs. This class is subdivided into two categories.

B1 – Cats diagnosed with left ventricular hypertrophy and mild left atrial enlargement.
B2 – Cats diagnosed with ventricular hypertrophy and moderate to severe left atrial enlargement.

Table 3.6 Summary of the feline classification system[1]

Stage	Description
A	Cats that are at risk of, or are predisposed to, developing cardiomyopathy but currently have no evidence of disease. This may be because of breed or familial history.
B	Cats in this group have been diagnosed with HCM (because they have increased left ventricular wall thickness) but importantly have no clinical signs. This group is divided in to two separate categories: B1 – Cats at **low risk** of developing congestive heart failure (CHF) or ATE imminently. This is because they have no or mild left atrial enlargement. B2 – Cats at **higher risk** of developing CHF or ATE imminently. This is because they have moderate to severe left atrial enlargement.
C	Cats that currently have, or have had, signs of CHF or an ATE.
D	Cats that have become refractory to conventional CHF treatment.

B1 – Diagnostic tests

- Although the majority of cats will not progress further than this stage, annual screening is recommended. This should include echocardiography and physical examination.

B1 – Nursing and treatment recommendations

- No treatment recommendations

B2 – Diagnostic tests

- It is recommended to monitor progress of the disease, but this should be weighed against the risk of stress to the cat. The use of pharmaceutical products, such as gabapentin may be prescribed, or synthetic feline pheromone products used, or both.
- Physical examination.
- Echocardiography – To assess left atrial size, left atrial appendage blood flow, presence of spontaneous echo contrast.
- Other diagnostic tests such as blood pressure and blood sampling to rule out concurrent diseases, such as hypertension, renal disease, and hyperthyroidism.

B2 – Nursing and treatment recommendations

- Cats must be handled carefully and stress minimised.
- Nurses can be proactive in advising owners how to bring their cats to the clinic, such as recommending synthetic feline pheromone products or the use of veterinary prescribed pharmaceuticals and appropriate carriers.
- Advise owners to count sleeping respiratory rate. This can help identify clinical signs developing.
- Clopidogrel (18.75 mg/cat PO once daily with food) is recommended for cats at risk of developing ATE. Other anti-thrombotics may also be considered in cats at high risk.
- For cats with ventricular arrhythmias, treatment with atenolol or sotalol may be recommended.

RECOMMENDATIONS OF NURSING AND TREATMENT OF STAGE C CATS

At this stage the cat has, or has had, clinical signs of heart failure or thromboembolism. This is a wide ranging group, including cats with chronic heart failure being managed on heart failure medication, to those in acute life-threatening heart failure. It also includes cats presenting with a thrombotic event, or those that have recovered.

Acute, life threatening heart failure – nursing and treatment

Cardiac emergencies are covered in more detail in Chapter 8.

- Furosemide (1–2 mg/kg) given either intramuscularly (IM) or intravenously (IV) if access can be achieved without stressing the cat further.
- The cat should be placed in a quiet environment with supplementary oxygen. A hiding place should be provided, but it should be possible to observe the cat without disturbing it.
- Gentle handling and minimise stress.

- If the cat is distressed, sedation may be appropriate. Butorphanol is recommended (0.2mg/kg).
- Prepare for thoracocentesis if pleural effusion is present.
- If the cat presents with low cardiac output, such as hypotension, hypothermia, or bradyarrhythmia, pimobendan may be considered (0.625–1.25 mg per cat q12h PO), if there is no outflow tract obstruction noted.
- If no improvement is noted with pimobendan, a continuous rate infusion of dobutamine might be considered. Continuous electrocardiography (ECG) should be attached and monitored and blood pressure measured regularly.
- It is recommended to send the cat home as soon as it has been stabilised, to minimise stress.
- The owner should be advised to monitor sleeping respiratory rate at home. The therapeutic goal is to maintain respiratory rate under 30 breaths/minute at home.

Re-examination is recommended three to seven days later to check for the resolution of heart failure, to assess renal function and electrolyte parameters, but this needs to be weighed against the stress of bringing the cat to the veterinary practice. A verbal or video update may be sufficient for anxious cats.

Chronic heart failure – Nursing and treatment recommendations

- Reducing stress is paramount, as cats can easily revert to life threatening heart failure.
- Administration of furosemide and clopidogrel if there is moderate to severe left atrial enlargement.
- After initiation of furosemide, it is recommended to re-examine the cat three to seven days later to check renal and electrolyte parameters.
- Pimobendan may be recommended to help contractility of the heart, as long as there is no outflow tract obstruction.
- Re-examination is recommended between 2 and 4 months, but the level of stress to the cat again needs to be considered. The presence of concurrent disease may warrant more frequent checks.
- Owner should monitor sleeping respiratory rate at home. The therapeutic goal is to maintain respiratory rate under 30 breaths/minute at home. Alterations in diuretic dose may be made over the telephone with the veterinary surgeon, according to the respiratory rate.

Management of aortic thromboembolism (ATE)

The most common treatment option is euthanasia when a cat presents at the clinic having experienced a thrombotic event[3], but if treatment is pursued, or if the owners need time to make a decision, the following recommendations have been made by the American College of Veterinary Internal Medicine consensus statement[1]. Cardiac emergencies are covered in more detail in Chapter 8.

Presentation – 24 hours post event

- Analgesia is crucial. The first 24 hours are considered the most painful, and recommendations are either methadone or fentanyl.
- Avoid stress.

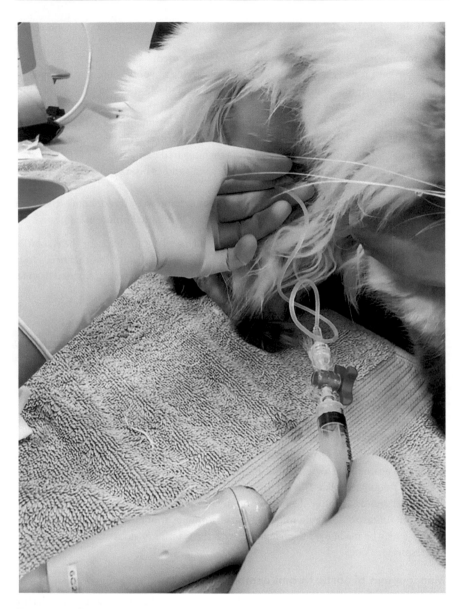

Figure 3.9 Thoracentesis in a cat.

- Anticoagulant therapy to be initiated as early as possible. Either low molecular weight heparin, unfractionated heparin, or an oral Xa inhibitor, if tolerated, such as rivaroxaban.
- If congestive heart failure is present, oxygen therapy and diuresis (either IM or IV) should be administered. However, pain can cause tachypnoea, and this should be taken into consideration.

- Check bedding, keep warm, and comfortable. Do not use direct heat sources to avoid scalds, room air is sufficient.
- Monitor vital signs, demeanour, mobility, renal function, and electrolytes.

24–72 Hours

- Assess pain and treat accordingly
- Monitor vital signs and for improvement of heart failure signs (if present)
- Monitor for azotaemia and possible reperfusion injury
- Monitor for local consequences of ischaemia, such as limb necrosis, self-mutilation, and limb contracture
- Physiotherapy may help, but use passive manipulation only
- Monitor urine output if hindlimb paralysis present

Post 72 Hours

- Go home with oral buprenorphine if necessary.
- Physiotherapy to be continued at home, if the cat is tolerating it. Owners should be shown how to perform passive manipulation.
- Communicate with the owner that deterioration or another event can occur.

Diagnostic tests

Tests should only be performed when the cat is stable enough to tolerate them. All diagnostic tests should be performed in as stress-free manner as possible, done in order of priority, and allowing the cat time to recover between each.

- Physical examination and auscultation. If pulmonary oedema is present, crackles may be heard over the lung fields. If pleural fluid is present, heart sounds (near the sternum) may sound muffled. Arrhythmias or a gallop rhythm may be heard and should be recorded. Efficacy of diuresis can be monitored by regular respiratory rate and effort.
- Blood pressure to assess cardiac output.
- Baseline laboratory tests, to include total protein and packed cell volume, creatinine, urea nitrogen, electrolytes, and urine specific gravity.
- Echocardiography can be used to confirm heart disease, measure chamber sizes, identify if spontaneous echo contrast or a thrombus is present, and to assess contractility of both the left ventricle and left atrium.

As echocardiography in cats can be challenging, a simple, focused point of care ultrasound examination may be used instead. By placing an ultrasound probe on the thorax, abnormal fluid can be detected (either pleural, pericardial or both), but also the presence of pulmonary oedema can be assessed by the presence of B lines (Figure 3.10), or to identify those cats at high risk of heart failure or ATE.

Radiography

Radiography is not particularly useful in diagnosing heart disease in cats. It is insensitive for mild to moderate cardiac changes, and the cardiac silhouette may look normal even in heart failure. Radiographs cannot identify phenotype, and the radiographic pattern of

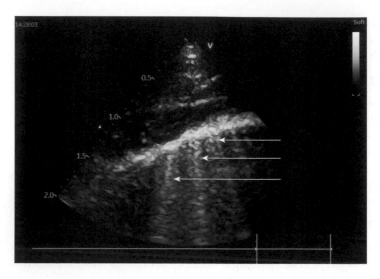

Figure 3.10 Image of B Lines on ultrasound.

pulmonary oedema is highly variable in cats. Given the lack or inconclusive information a radiograph can provide, it needs to be considered how safe a diagnostic test is for the cat. If the cat is tachypnoeic or in respiratory distress, compromising its lung function by placing it in lateral recumbency for a radiograph is contraindicated.

Biomarkers

Biomarkers also have limited use in helping diagnose feline heart disease. N-Terminal pro B-type natriuretic peptide (NTproBNP) can distinguish between respiratory and cardiac dyspnoea, but is not useful for mild to moderate disease. Cardiac troponin I (cTnI) also distinguishes between respiratory and cardiac dyspnoea, but also has been shown to be an independent predicator of cardiac death, separate from left atrial size. Current advice is to use a combination of a biomarker and other tests to diagnose HCM.

RECOMMENDATIONS OF NURSING AND TREATMENT OF STAGE D CATS

Patients that are classified at stage D are not responding to standard heart failure medication. As with stage C patients, class D patients can also present in acute, life-threatening heart failure or chronic heart failure.

Acute and life-threatening refractory heart failure – Nursing and treatment recommendations

Very similar nursing and treatment aims to class C acute heart failure patients, in that stress must be avoided and oxygen supplementation may be necessary. Torasemide (at a starting dose of 0.1–0.2 mg/kg per os once daily) may replace furosemide as the diuretic of choice. Other additional medications may be added at this stage, such as spironolactone (1–2 mg/kg per os either once or twice daily), potassium supplementation, or pimobendan (0.625–1.25 mg per cat per os once daily) if it has not been prescribed already. Nursing actions include:

- Minimising stress and providing oxygen supplementation.
- Good client communication. Owner compliance may decrease with the addition of medication.

Diagnostic tests

Same as class C

Chronic refractory heart failure – Nursing and treatment recommendations

Cats with chronic refractory heart failure will require the same nursing and treatment as cats in class C. Key points include

- Good client communication and support is vital. Owner to monitor resting respiratory rate at home.
- Body weight and body condition score should be monitored.
- Cardiac cachexia can be present in stage D. If it is, calorie intake should be prioritised over sodium restriction.

PROGNOSIS OF HEART DISEASE AND HEART FAILURE

Not all cats diagnosed with cardiomyopathy will progress to heart failure, and some live unaffected lives. For example, some cats with focal left ventricular hypertrophy tolerate it well. When a cat has been diagnosed with heart failure resulting from their heart disease, prognosis can still vary, and will depend upon whether the owner can medicate their cat. Negative prognostic indicators on echocardiography include limited left atrial function, extreme left ventricular hypertrophy and restricted left ventricular systolic function.

PROGNOSIS FOR ATE

There are a number of indicators that point to a poor prognosis. For example, low rectal temperature, two or more affected limbs, concurrent heart failure, bradycardia, lack of motor function, and hyperphosphataemia are negative prognostic indicators. Recurrence is common. As with heart failure, survival time is also dependent upon whether the owner can medicate their cat.

KEY POINTS

- HCM is the most common form of feline cardiomyopathy, but the prevalence of other phenotypes is not known.
- Approximately a third of cats aged over nine could have heart disease.
- ATE occurs as a result of heart disease, and prognosis is poor.
- Oxygen supplementation and minimising stress are crucial nursing actions.

FURTHER READING

Luis Fuentes V, Abbott J, Chetboul V, Côté E, Fox PR, Häggström J, Kittleson MD, Schober K, Stern JA (2020). ACVIM consensus statement guidelines for the classification, diagnosis, and management of cardiomyopathies in cats. *Journal of Veterinary Internal Medicine*. 34(3): 1062–1077.

Borgeat K, Wright J, Garrod O, Payne JR, Luis Fuentes V (2014). Arterial thromboembolism in 250 cats in general practice: 2004–2012. *Journal of Veterinary Internal Medicine*. 28: 102–108.

REFERENCES

1. Luis Fuentes V, Abbott J, Chetboul V, Côté E, Fox PR, Häggström J, Kittleson MD, Schober K, Stern JA (2020). ACVIM consensus statement guidelines for the classification, diagnosis, and management of cardiomyopathies in cats. *Journal of Veterinary Internal Medicine*. 34(3): 1062–1077.
2. Payne JR, Brodbelt DC, Luis Fuentes V (2015). Cardiomyopathy prevalence in 780 apparently healthy cats in rehoming centres (The CatScan Study). *Journal Veterinary Cardiology*. Dec;17 Suppl 1: S244–57. https://doi.org/10.1016/j.jvc.2015.03.008.
3. Borgeat K, Wright J, Garrod O, Payne JR, Luis Fuentes V (2014). Arterial thromboembolism in 250 cats in general practice: 2004–2012. *Journal of Veterinary Internal Medicine*. 28: 102–108.
4. Wagner T, Luis Fuentes V, Payne JR, McDermott N, Brodbelt D (2010). Comparison of auscultatory and echocardiographic findings in healthy adult cats. *Journal of Veterinary Cardiology*. Dec;12(3):171–82. https://doi.org/10.1016/j.jvc.2010.05.003.

Congenital heart disease

Congenital heart disease (CHD) is either a malformation of one or more areas of the heart or the great vessels (aorta or pulmonary artery) or the persistence of a normal foetal structure following birth. CHD is relatively uncommon in general practice, but an awareness of the more common diseases is useful. Studies have shown that the prevalence of CHD in cats in the general population is between 0.02% and 0.1% and in dogs between 0.5% and 1.0%[1]. This chapter looks at the most common diseases and classified into the type of heart failure they can cause. Table 4.1 shows the most common congenital diseases diagnosed in dogs and cats, by order of prevalence.

ASYMPTOMATIC CHD

Ventricular septal defect (VSD)

A ventricular septal defect (VSD) is a hole in the intraventricular septal wall. It is usually found in the membranous part of the septum, just below the aortic valve. Due to the higher pressures in the left ventricle, blood usually flows from the left side to right. It is this shunting of blood that causes the murmur. A smaller defect offers more resistance to blood flow, and therefore creates a louder murmur. A larger hole offers less resistance, resulting in a quieter murmur. Figure 4.1 illustrates a VSD, and 4.2 shows a VSD as seen on echocardiography.

A left sided systolic heart murmur is usually detected at first vaccination, and most animals do not have any clinical signs. Patients with large VSDs may experience left sided congestive heart failure (L-CHF). Treatment is not recommended in small VSDs.

Diseases causing left sided congestive heart failure (L-CHF)

See Chapter 1 for clinical signs of L-CHF.

Patent ductus arteriosus (PDA)

A patent ductus arteriosus (PDA) is a CHD where the normal ductal arteriosus has failed to close after birth. In utero, the ductus arteriosus connects the aorta and the pulmonary artery, where it takes blood away from the heart because the lungs are not used. At birth, several factors should close the ductus. However, in some rare cases, the ductus arteriosus remains open. Intracardiac pressure in the aorta is greater than in the pulmonary artery,

DOI: 10.1201/9781003122173-5

Table 4.1 Most common CHD reported in dogs and cats in order of prevalence

Dogs	Cats
Pulmonic stenosis	Ventricular septal defect
Patent ductus arteriosus	Aortic stenosis
Aortic stenosis	Hypertrophic obstructive cardiomyopathy
Ventricular septal defect	Pulmonic stenosis

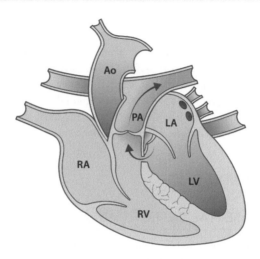

Figure 4.1 Picture of a VSD. Note how oxygenated blood from the left ventricle crosses the hole and flows into the pulmonary artery, mixing with deoxygenated blood. Ao = Aorta. Pa = Pulmonary artery. LA = left atrium. LV = Left ventricle. RA = Right atrium. RV = Right ventricle.

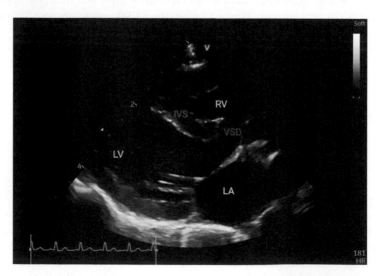

Figure 4.2 VSD on echo. IVS = Intraventricular septum, RV = right ventricle. RV = Right ventricle. LV = Left ventricle. IVS = Intraventricular septum. LA = Left atrium.

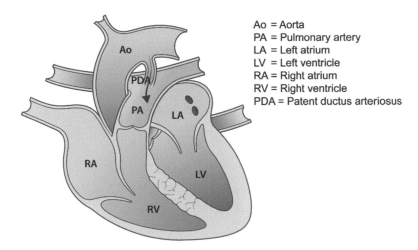

Ao = Aorta
PA = Pulmonary artery
LA = Left atrium
LV = Left ventricle
RA = Right atrium
RV = Right ventricle
PDA = Patent ductus arteriosus

Figure 4.3 Picture of a PDA.

and so blood shunts across the PDA continuously. This can create volume overload of the left heart, causing L-CHF. Figure 4.3 shows a PDA and how blood flow moves from the aorta to the pulmonary artery. Figure 4.4 highlights a PDA on echocardiography, and 4.5 shows a canine ductal occluder, used to close a PDA.

There appears to be a breed predisposition including German Shepherd Dogs, Shetland Sheepdogs, English Springer Spaniels, Bichon Frise, Poodles, and Yorkshire Terriers. A greater number of dogs are female. Cats can also be diagnosed with PDA, but it is less common.

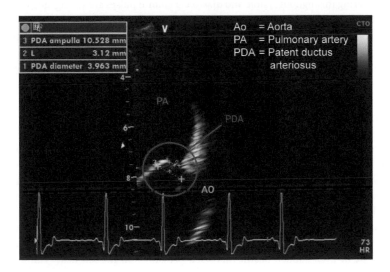

Figure 4.4 PDA seen on echocardiography. Note how the ductus arteriousus is open. This should normally close at or around birth. The measurements allow for an appropriate-sized ductal occluder to be placed to close the ductus.

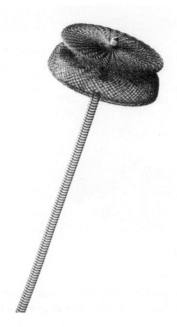

Figure 4.5 An Amplatz canine ductal occluder. Image courtesy Infiniti Medical LLC, Palo Alto, CA USA. This is placed via the femoral artery into the PDA, to close the ductus.

A loud heart murmur, often accompanied with a palpable thrill (either grade V/VI or VI/VI) is usually detected at first vaccination. It is a distinct murmur because it is continuous, occurring throughout systole and diastole. Femoral pulses are strong and jerky. Many dogs will present cachexic. Diagnosis can be confirmed with echocardiography, which can also be used to rule out any other cardiac abnormalities. Treatment options are available, such as using a device to plug the ductus using interventional cardiograhic techniques, or surgical ligation of the vessel. If the patient is treated young enough, a good prognosis is possible, and a full recovery made. If signs of L-CHF are present, these need to be treated.

Aortic stenosis (AS)

AS occurs where there is a narrowing of the aorta. It has been recognised to have three forms, valvular, subvalvular, and rarely, supravalvular. Subvalvular AS is the most common type, where protruding lesions usually consist of fibrous bands. The stenosis can vary from a small lesion of little clinical significance to a concentric band causing severe clinical signs. The stenosis causes an obstruction to blood flow leaving the left ventricle, and myocardial hypertrophy can occur as the ventricle works harder to eject blood. The increased stress on the ventricular wall can cause ventricular arrhythmias, leading to syncope or even sudden death. Increased pressures on the left heart can also cause L-CHF. Figure 4.6 shows aortic stenosis in diagrammatic form.

Breeds with a predilection to AS are Boxers, Golden Retrievers, German Shepherd Dogs, and Newfoundlands. AS can be diagnosed in cats also, but can be difficult

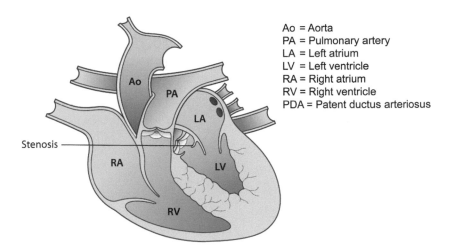

Ao = Aorta
PA = Pulmonary artery
LA = Left atrium
LV = Left ventricle
RA = Right atrium
RV = Right ventricle
PDA = Patent ductus arteriosus

Figure 4.6 Picture of AS.

to differentiate from left ventricular hypertrophy due to outflow obstruction or the hypertrophy cardiomyopathy phenotype. The main difference seems to be age of presentation.

A left sided systolic murmur at the heart base is often auscultated at first vaccination, or a patient may present with clinical signs such as exercise intolerance or syncope. Diagnosis is confirmed by echocardiography. Clinical signs will vary on the severity of the stenosis, and some patients may be asymptomatic. Most cases are mild to moderate and will not require treatment, but in some cases interventional cardiology or surgical correction may be possible. Medical management may include treatment for heart failure or beta blockade to reduce myocardial oxygen consumption.

RIGHT SIDED CONGESTIVE HEART FAILURE (R-CHF)

See Chapter 1 for clinical signs of R-CHF.

PULMONIC STENOSIS (PS)

PS is a narrowing of the pulmonic artery. Similar to AS, stenosis can occur below or above the valve, but in contrast, the most common type is valvular stenosis. PS can lead to right ventricular hypertrophy, and in severe cases, cause R-CHF. Figure 4.7 shows pulmonic stenosis in diagrammatic form.

Breeds predisposed to PS are Boxers, Beagles, Cocker Spaniels, Miniature Schnauzer, English Bulldog, and terriers. PS can be seen in cats, often with other congenital cardiac defects. A left sided systolic murmur at the heart base is often auscultated at first vaccination, or a patient may present with clinical signs such as exercise intolerance or syncope. Diagnosis is confirmed with echocardiography. As with AS, clinical signs will vary on the severity of the stenosis, and some patients may be asymptomatic. The majority of cases are

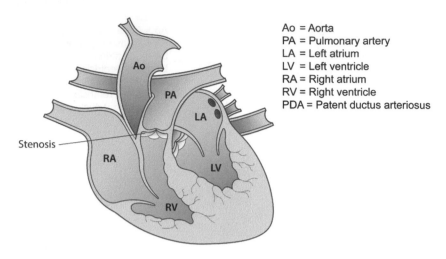

Ao = Aorta
PA = Pulmonary artery
LA = Left atrium
LV = Left ventricle
RA = Right atrium
RV = Right ventricle
PDA = Patent ductus arteriosus

Figure 4.7 Picture of PS.

mild and do not require treatment. Medical management may include treatment for heart failure or beta blockade to reduce myocardial oxygen consumption. Severe cases of PS may benefit from balloon valvuloplasty, if valvular stenosis is present. Surgical intervention can also be considered. Figure 4.8(a and b) shows a balloon valvuloplasty where the stenosis is 'burst' by a balloon catheter.

CYANOTIC CHD

TETRALOGY OF FALLOT (ToF)

Tetralogy of Fallot (ToF) is a rare cardiac disorder, but it is the most common of the cyanotic congenital defects. Figure 4.9 illustrates the defects making a ToF, and 4.10 shows ToF on echocardiography. It comprises of four different defects:

- *Pulmonic stenosis* – The pulmonary artery is either narrowed or hypoplastic (underdeveloped)
- *Overriding aorta* – The aorta is wide and displaced
- *Large ventricular septal defect* – Due to malalignment of the intraventricular septum
- *Right ventricular hypertrophy* – Increased pressure on the right ventricle because of the pulmonic stenosis

Patients usually present with stunted growth, severe exercise intolerance and cyanosis of the mucous membranes. Due to the high pressure in the right ventricle because of the PS, blood freely shunts across the VSD into the left ventricle. This mixes oxygenated blood with deoxygenated blood, which is then ejected into the systemic circulation via the aorta. This causes hypoxemia, which the body tries to compensate for, by increasing red cell production, causing marked polycythaemia.

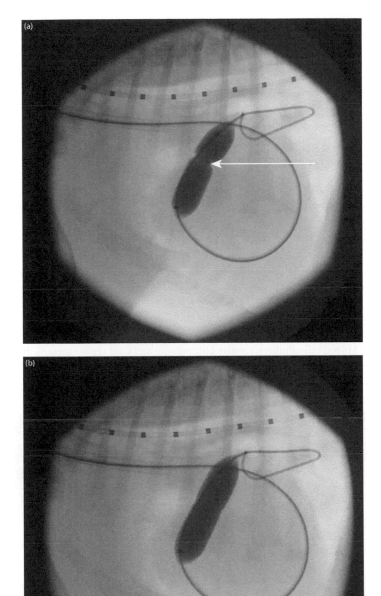

Figure 4.8 (a) Fluoroscopy image showing balloon catheter across the pulmonic valve. The waist indicates the stenosis. And (b) fluoroscopy image showing the waist has gone.

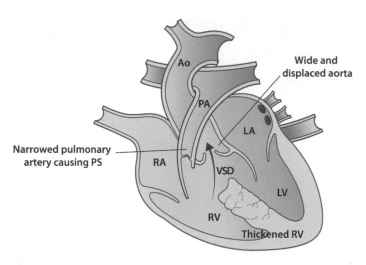

Figure 4.9 Picture of Tetralogy of Fallot. Note how deoxygenated and oxygenated blood mix in the aorta due to the VSD.

The severity of clinical signs varies on the degree of the defects. Medical treatment may include beta blockade to minimise myocardial oxygen demand, hydroxyurea to reduce red blood cell numbers, regular phlebotomy and fluid replacement to dilute blood viscosity. When performing phlebotomy, a target PCV of 60%–65% should be aimed at. Surgical intervention can be attempted, but is only palliative.

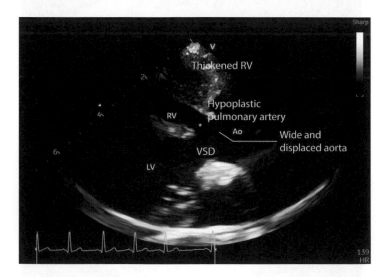

Figure 4.10 Part of ToF visible on echocardiography. Note in this picture, the right ventricular hypertrophy (labelled), the VSD allowing communication of the left and right ventricles, and the wide aorta (labelled). It is easy to see how oxygenated and deoxygenated blood are mixed and leave through the aorta. RV = Right ventricle. Ao = Aorta. LV = Left ventricle. VSD = ventricular septal defect.

KEY POINTS

- CHD is rare in small animal practice
- Clinical signs and prognosis vary depending upon the severity of the defect(s)

FURTHER READING

1. Martin M, Dukes-McEwan J (2010). Congenital heart disease. In: *BSAVA Manual of Canine and Feline Cardiorespiratory Medicine*, 2nd edition. British Small Animal Veterinary Association, Gloucester.

5

Electrocardiography

An electrocardiograph (ECG) can be a vital diagnostic tool in determining heart rate and heart rhythm. There are many reasons that attaching an ECG might be beneficial, such as monitoring anaesthesia and for emergency case management. This chapter will discuss the machine and its settings, describe how to create a good quality ECG trace and some basic steps for interpretation, and then provide some information on common arrhythmias. The conduction system is described in Chapter 1.

THE MACHINE

There are many different makes and models of ECG machines available. Some machines used in practice were originally designed for use in human medicine, and some machines have been designed specifically for the veterinary market. Some machines are stand-alone ECG machines, but most practices have multiparameter ECG machines, capable of recording oxygen saturation, exhaled carbon dioxide, blood pressure, and temperature simultaneously. Some machines are completely digital, some older versions are paper only, and some have capacity to store digitally and print. Figure 5.1 shows an example of an ECG machine, and Table 5.1 summarises terminology used.

ELECTRODES

Electrodes are the point of contact to the body surface (Figure 5.2). Standard protocol for exact measurements, suggest that the electrodes should be placed behind the elbows and in front of the stifles, but this may not always be possible. For example, a cat may have an intravenous catheter bandage, or a patient is missing a leg, or in surgery if the patient is too long for the cables. A more practical solution is the general principle that the electrodes should create a triangle around the heart, which means that the flank may be preferable in a large dog under anaesthesia.

Old fashioned machines use crocodile clips, but preference is now for atraumatic clips as seen in Figure 5.2. Other types of electrodes available are adhesive pads placed on the feet, which are particularly useful for surgery, because they are securely attached. To allow for good contact, a conduction agent is needed, which can either be electrical coupling gel or ultrasound gel, or a small amount of surgical spirit. Surgical spirit requires no cleaning, and is fast to provide a trace, but is flammable, so should be used with caution, if defibrillation may be required. If in doubt, conduction gel should be used.

DOI: 10.1201/9781003122173-6

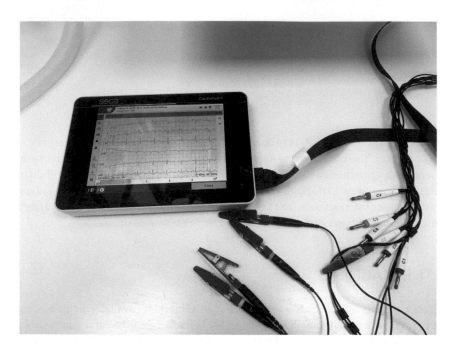

Figure 5.1 Picture of digital ECG machine with electrodes and cables. (Photo courtesy of Paul Smith.)

The electrodes need to be placed in a specific order, but manufacturing guidelines vary in different countries, and colours can differ. Table 5.2 shows the two main colour schemes. If in doubt, refer to the machine's manual for clarification.

CABLES

The cables are the wires that connect the patient to the ECG machine. For a good quality trace, they should be untangled, and attached to the electrodes without touching each other. The cables should always come away from the patient, not crossing the thorax, as breathing, movement and/or muscle tremor can cause artefact to occur. Figure 5.3 shows gold standard positioning, with the cables labelled.

The number of cables can vary, depending upon the machine. Some machines have three cables, some four, five, six, or twelve. Standard machines consist of four cables and electrodes. The difference between three and four cables is in how the trace is viewed. An

Table 5.1 Terminology

Electrodes = Point of contact at the body surface
Cables = Wires connecting the electrodes to the machine
Leads = ECG trace created from the electrodes attached to the body

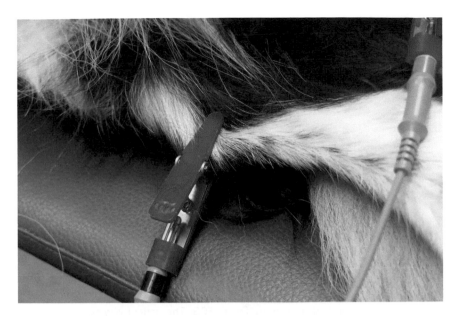

Figure 5.2 Picture of electrodes. Newer versions of crocodile clips have smooth edges and are tolerated much better by conscious patients. (Photo courtesy of Paul Smith.)

ECG trace is created by forming a triangle around the heart, using one electrode as an earth (Figure 5.4). If there are three cables and one is acting as the earth, then the trace can only be viewed in one lead (like most multiparameter machines). However, if there are four cables, then all the leads creating the triangle can be viewed at the same time, displaying leads I, II, and III. If the ECG machine has the capacity, then the three electrodes can translate to a six lead trace, leads I, II, III and aVR, aVF, and aVL (Figure 5.5). The six lead ECG allows for a more detailed interpretation, as each lead has a different perspective of the heart. Six leads are most commonly used by cardiologists, who use it to investigate conduction abnormalities or chamber enlargement.

LEADS

The leads are the ECG trace created from the electrodes attached to the body. The most common lead to interpret is lead II, as indicated in Figure 5.6.

Table 5.2 Electrode placement

United Kingdom/European	United States of America
Red = right forelimb	White = right forelimb
Yellow = left forelimb	Black = left forelimb
Green = left hindlimb	Red = left hindlimb
Black lead = right hindlimb	Green lead = right hindlimb

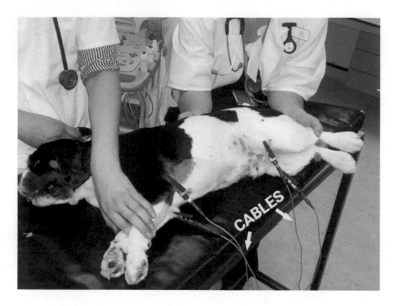

Figure 5.3 Gold standard positioning for an ECG. The patient is lying in right lateral recumbency, on a non-conductive comfortable surface (a vetbed is sufficient), with the limbs separated and cables running away from the patient.

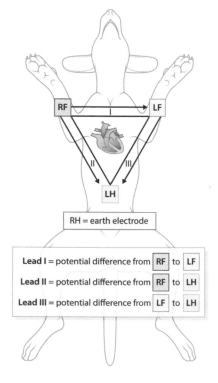

RF = earth electrode

Lead I = potential difference from RF to LF

Lead II = potential difference from RF to LH

Lead III = potential difference from LF to LH

Figure 5.4 How the ECG leads form a triangle around the heart and become a three lead trace.

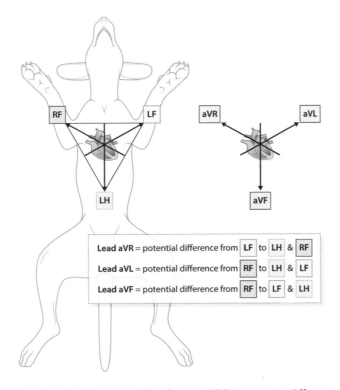

Lead aVR = potential difference from	LF	to	LH	&	RF
Lead aVL = potential difference from	RF	to	LH	&	LF
Lead aVF = potential difference from	RF	to	LF	&	LH

Figure 5.5 How three leads become six leads on an ECG trace, using different viewpoints.

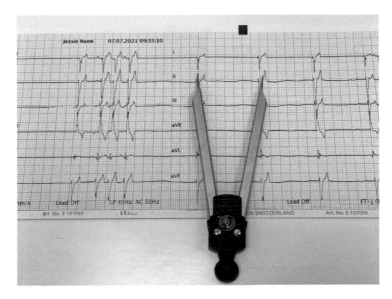

Figure 5.6 This is a six lead ECG trace. The placement of four electrodes and cables allows this ECG trace to be seen in all six leads. Interpretation occurs in lead II most commonly. (Photo courtesy of Paul Smith.)

Machine settings

- *Leads and display screens* – Most modern ECG machines have a display screen. Some displays will show leads I–III, but some, like multiparameter machines for example, can only show one lead at a time. Some machines will show leads I–III and aVR, aVF, and aVL. Lead II is the main lead used for interpretation, so if only one lead can be shown, it should be lead II.
- *Filter* – Most machines have a filter switch. The advantage is that having a filter on can dampen artefact making interpretation easier, but in cats, a filter can dampen so much that P waves can be eliminated as interference.
- *Paper speed* – There are usually two speeds available, 25 mm/second and 50 mm/second. 50 mm/second makes the paper speed faster, which spreads out the complexes more, making interpretation easier. This can be useful when looking for P waves in fast rhythms.
- *Sensitivity* – Sensitivity makes the complexes either bigger or smaller. The larger the number, the bigger the complexes. It is recommended to start with 10 mV, and adjust as necessary.

Artefact

Artefact is interference on the ECG trace that can hamper diagnosis. Efforts should be made to minimise it, for example keeping the patient as calm as possible, performing the ECG in a quiet place, and switching off unnecessary electrical equipment. Table 5.3 lists

Table 5.3 Component parts of the sinus complex

P wave	The sinoatrial (SA) node starts the depolarisation process. The electrical impulse spreads from right to left across the atria. When the whole of the atria have been depolarised, the electrical difference returns to baseline.
P–R interval	The atrioventricular (AV) node slowly conducts the impulse from the atria to the ventricles to allow for coordinated ventricular contraction. No muscle is depolarised, therefore the baseline remains flat.
Q Wave	Depolarisation of the ventricular septum.
R Wave	The large muscle mass of the ventricles is depolarised via the His-Purkinje fibre network.
S Wave	The remaining basal regions of the ventricles are depolarised.
T Wave	Repolarisation of the ventricles, so they are ready to start the process again. T wave morphology can vary largely from patient to patient, and are generally not of diagnostic value in small animal medicine.

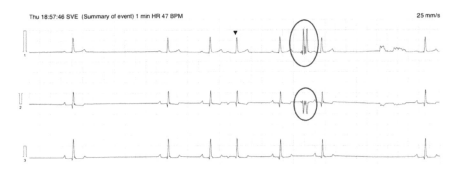

Thu 18:57:46 SVE (Summary of event) 1 min HR 47 BPM   25 mm/s

Figure 5.7 Artefact in leads I and II, caused by movement. Red circles highlight interference.

possible causes of artefact. Figure 5.7 shows movement artefact and 5.8 illustrates purring artefact on lead II.

Electrical – Such as fans or clippers
Panting
Muscle tremor
Patient movement
Purring

POSITIONING

Along with correct electrode placement, positioning is also important. The standard position is right lateral recumbency, with the patient lying on a vetbed or non-conductive surface. Ideally, the electrodes should be attached behind the elbows and in front of the stifles. The cables untangled, not touching, and run away from the patient, to minimise

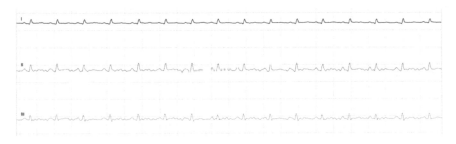

Figure 5.8 Purring artefact. Note the difficulty in distinguishing P waves from movement on lead II.

artefact interference. The patient should be as calm as possible, and unless investigating the side effect of drugs, be taken before sedation or premedication is administered. Figure 5.3 shows correct positioning.

For patients that do not tolerate lateral recumbency, for cats, and any patient in respiratory distress, sternal recumbency is recommended. If working with a cardiology specialist, it is advisable to tell them the recording was recorded in sternal, as this may make minor differences to measurements.

REASONS FOR PERFORMING AN ECG

Recording an ECG is a vital part of monitoring patients in a number of situations. Below are some of the reasons why an ECG may be required.

- Anaesthesia
- Emergencies
- Post-surgical cases
- If an arrhythmia is suspected on auscultation or history
- Drug toxicity
- Electrolyte disturbances
- To assess effectiveness of cardiac drugs

TIPS TO PERFORMING A GOOD QUALITY ECG AND TROUBLESHOOTING GUIDE

Box 5.1 provides a simple trouble shooting guide, if obtaining a good quality trace is problematic.

BOX 5.1: How to ensure a good ECG trace is recorded

EQUIPMENT

Have machine ready for use, and on correct settings, before attaching to the
 patient
Have conduction agent available
Cables untangled, ready for use
Electrodes ready. If using crocodile/atraumatic clips, these can be attached to the
 cables in preparation.
Prepare vetbed

PATIENT

Patient as calm as possible, lying in right lateral recumbency
If patient is in respiratory distress, or scared, position in sternal recumbency
Attach electrodes and apply conducting agent, ensuring that they do not touch
Ensure lead II is selected/visible and record trace
Cats – Prioritise 50 mm/second using a sensitivity of at least 10 mV

TROUBLE SHOOTING

Poor quality trace

- Replace electrodes and apply more conductive agent (either surgical spirit or gel).
- Consider what the veterinary surgeon is doing. Are the cables moving? If so, either wait and see if it settles, or tell them.
- Or are the cables across the thorax and the trace is being moved by respiration?

One line missing on the display screen

- Replace electrodes and apply more conductive agent (either surgical spirit or gel)

Recording a cat ECG and the trace is too small

- Change the sensitivity. Select sensitivity. Bigger the number, bigger the complex.

Recording a dog ECG and the trace is too big

- Change the sensitivity. Select sensitivity. Smaller the number, smaller the complex.

The complexes need to be spaced out more

- Change the paper speed. 50 mm/second spaces out the complexes more

INTERPRETATION

It is useful if nurses can not only take a reliable ECG, but also be able to interpret it, so they can seek veterinary surgeon assistance promptly when required. The anatomy and function of the conduction system is discussed in Chapter 1. The conduction system is shown in Figure 5.9. This chapter focuses on the trace produced. The standard lead of interpretation is lead II, and the normal, or sinus, complex should look similar to Figure 5.10, with a P-QRS-T wave.

Each part of the sinus complex correlates to electrical activity, and is broken down in Table 5.3.

INTERPRETATION GUIDE

Recognising sinus rhythms is important because it is easier to recognise when things are not right. A simple five step guide can help interpretation.

1. What is the heart rate?
2. Is there a P wave for every QRS?

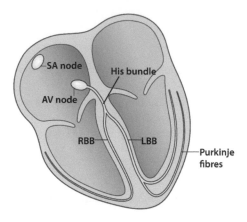

Figure 5.9 Labelled diagram of the conduction system.

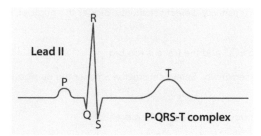

Figure 5.10 Labelled diagram of a sinus complex. SA = Sinoatrial node. AV = Atrioventricular node. LBB = Left bundle branch. RBB = Right bundle branch.

3. Is there a Q wave for every P?
4. Are they reasonably and consistently related?
5. What is the morphology (shape) of the QRS wave? Tall and narrow, or wide and bizarre?

QUESTION 1 – WHAT IS THE HEART RATE?

Life threatening rhythms are usually very fast or very slow; therefore, determining the heart rate is an important first step. Some machines record heart rate automatically, but machines can double count complexes, or be unreliable when heart rate is variable, such as a ventricular run in an otherwise sinus rhythm. Table 5.4 shows expected ranges for heart rates.

To calculate the heart rate, on a paper copy of the ECG trace, either:

• Use an ECG ruler. One side is marked for 25 mm/second (Figure 5.11), and the reverse for 50 mm/second (Figure 5.12).

    or

• Measure a 6 second interval (15 cm at a paper speed of 25 mm/second or 30 cm at a paper speed of 50 mm/second) and count the number of QRS complexes within this period. Multiply by ten to reach number of beats per minute.

Understanding the heart rate can help narrow down the possible arrhythmia choice. Figure 5.13 shows the possible rhythms associated with heart rate.

Table 5.4 Expected heart rates

Adult dog	70–160 beats/minute
Giant breeds	60–140 beats/minute
Toy breeds	70–180 beats/minute
Puppies	70–220 beats/minute
Adult cats	120–240 beats/minute

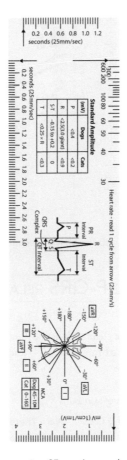

Figure 5.11 Shows ECG ruler measuring 25 mm/second.

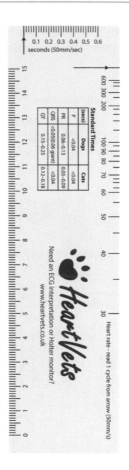

Figure 5.12 Shows ECG ruler measuring 50 mm/second.

QUESTIONS 2–4: THE P-QRS RELATIONSHIP

QUESTION 2 – IS THERE A P WAVE FOR EVERY QRS?

Each sinus complex should have a clear and visible P wave and a QRS wave accompanying it. If there is not, consider the heart rate (Table 5.4) and compare to the possible arrhythmias in Figure 5.14 and Table 5.5.

Table 5.5 Possible answers for Question 2

Yes – There is a P wave for every QRS	No – There is not a P wave for every QRS
Are they consistently and reasonably related? See Question 4	Atrial fibrillation Atrial standstill Ventricular tachycardia Premature complexes (atrial or ventricular) Escape complexes

QUESTION 3 – IS THERE A QRS COMPLEX FOR EVERY P WAVE?

Each sinus complex should have a QRS wave and P wave preceding it. If there is not, consider the heart rate (Table 5.4) and compare to the possible arrhythmias in Figures 5.13 and 5.14 and Table 5.6.

Table 5.6 Possible answers for Question 3

Yes – There is a QRS complex for every P wave	No – There is not a QRS complex for every P wave
Are they consistently and reasonably related? See Question 4	2nd degree AV block 3rd degree AV block Atrial flutter

QUESTION 4 – ARE THEY CONSISTENTLY AND REASONABLY RELATED?

To enable normal conduction, the sinus rhythm requires the P-QRS to be consistently, and obviously related to each other. If there is not this consistency, consider the heart rate (Table 5.4 and Figure 5.13) and compare the possible arrhythmias in Figure 5.14 and Table 5.7.

Table 5.7 Possible answers for Question 4

Yes – The P waves and QRS complexes are consistently related to each other	No – The P waves and QRS complexes are not consistently related to each other
Sinus rhythm Sinus arrhythmia Sinus bradycardia Atrial premature complexes	3rd degree AV block Ventricular tachycardia

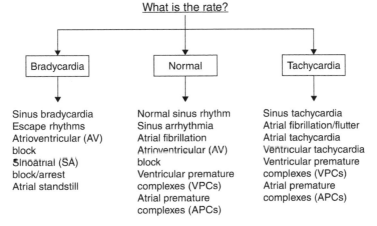

Figure 5.13 Following this simple heart rate algorithm can help narrow down arrhythmia possibilities.

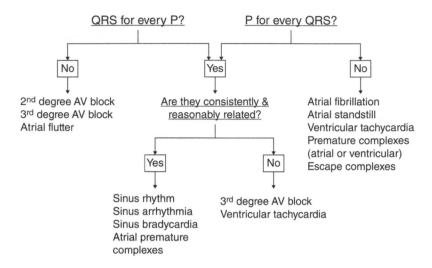

Figure 5.14 Summary of Questions 2–4.

QUESTION 5 – WHAT IS THE MORPHOLOGY (SHAPE) OF THE QRS WAVE? TALL AND NARROW, OR WIDE AND BIZARRE?

The sinus complex should originate within the atria, and therefore the impulse uses the conduction system, quickly and efficiently, thereby producing a narrow complex. If the impulse has originated in the ventricles however, the QRS complex will generally be wide and bizarre, because it has had to depolarise the myocardium cell by cell. This takes longer, and therefore, the complex appears wide and bizarre (Figure 5.15). Figure 5.16 shows an example of an atrial premature complex. The impulse has originated in the atrium, so it is tall and narrow, but lacks a P wave.

The one main exception to this can be the appearance of cat sinus complexes on ECG. It is a common finding especially in older cats either with or without heart disease, and it is called left anterior fascicular block (Figure 5.17). It is a normal sinus complex, with a P-QRS wave, but the QRS complex is abnormal in its direction. It does not cause clinical

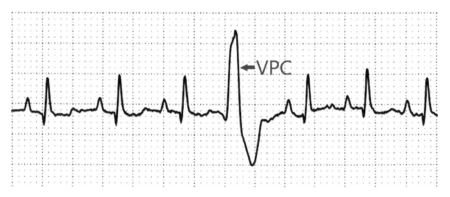

Figure 5.15 Example of a wide and bizarre complex in an otherwise sinus rhythm. Note the lack of a P wave and how different the complex looks compared to a sinus complex. This is a ventricular premature complex (VPC).

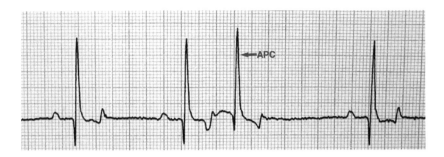

Figure 5.16 Example of tall and narrow complex in an otherwise sinus rhythm. Note the lack of a P wave and how different the complex looks compared to a sinus complex. This is an atrial or supraventricular premature complex (APC).

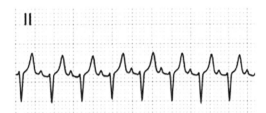

Figure 5.17 Example of left anterior fascicular block in a cat. Note the normal sinus rhythm, but that the QRS complexes are wide.

signs in itself, and is a result of a failure of conduction through the anterior fascicle of the left bundle branch.

SINUS RHYTHMS

The appearance of a sinus complex is individual to each patient, so after determining the rate, it is important to assess whether each complex has a P-QRS for each and every complex, and to assess what is normal for the individual patient. On auscultation of sinus rhythms, the normal 'lub dub' heart sounds can be heard. Figure 5.18 shows a sinus rhythm in a dog.

Because cat hearts are smaller, the complexes will be smaller. It may be necessary to increase the amplitude of the waves by increasing the sensitivity, to identify P waves clearly. It is especially important therefore, to minimise artefact when recording. Figure 5.19 shows the smaller complex size with a cat sinus rhythm.

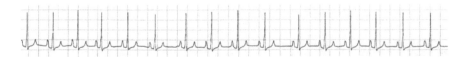

Figure 5.18 Sinus rhythm in a dog.

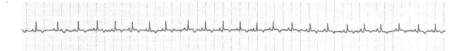

Figure 5.19 Sinus rhythm in a cat.

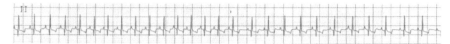

Figure 5.20 Sinus tachycardia in a dog. Heart rate is 180 beats/minute.

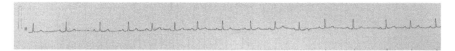

Figure 5.21 Sinus bradycardia in a cat. Heart rate is 80 beats/minute.

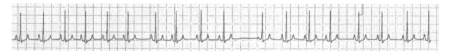

Figure 5.22 Sinus arrhythmia. Note the uneven intervals between QRS complexes.

SINUS TACHYCARDIA

A normal rhythm with a P wave for every QRS complex that is faster than normal for the age and breed of the animal (Figure 5.20). It can be a normal finding in dogs and cats, and be a response to pain, fear or excitement. There is a pulse with every heartbeat.

SINUS BRADYCARDIA

A normal rhythm with a P wave for every QRS complex that is slower than normal for the age and breed of the animal. It is often seen in giant breed dogs, but also in athletic or working dogs. There is a pulse with every heartbeat. Figure 5.21 is an example of sinus bradycardia in a cat.

SINUS ARRHYTHMIA

A rhythm that has a P-QRS wave, but the heart rate varies. It is a normal and common finding in dogs, often linked with respiration, and known as respiratory sinus arrhythmia. It is associated with increased vagal tone, but is uncommon in cats. An example of sinus arrhythmia can be seen in Figure 5.22.

COMMON ARRHYTHMIAS

Arrhythmias can occur for many different reasons, either related to cardiac disease or not. In dogs, arrhythmias are most commonly seen with non-cardiac disease, but with

---

BOX 5.2: Common causes of arrhythmias. This list is by no means exhaustive

Structural heart disease

Hypoxia

Inflammation or inflammatory diseases

Autonomic imbalance

Metabolic abnormalities, such as hyperkalaemia

Drugs

Toxins

Temperature – Either hyper or hypothermia

---

cats, arrhythmias are more commonly associated with heart disease. Box 5.2 lists some of the common causes of arrhythmias seen in small animal practice. Some arrhythmias can be life threatening, and this is where a basic understanding of cardiac physiology can help. When the heart works as it should, haemodynamic stability is maintained. As with heart disease, electrical conduction can compromise cardiac output. The formula cardiac output = heart rate + stroke volume is once again useful here.

If the heart rate is consistently too fast, cardiac output can be compromised, because the ventricles need time to relax and refill with blood in diastole. This is vital to maintain blood pressure and blood supply to the rest of the body, but also to supply the heart itself. If the heart cannot maintain coronary perfusion, this can promote further arrhythmias. Equally, prolonged periods of very slow rates can also affect cardiac output.

Another problem with arrhythmias is that as well as being haemodynamically unstable, they can also be electrically unstable. For example, if the heart does not have long enough to refill and perfuse itself, seen in some cases of ventricular tachycardia, the heart may attempt to work even harder to compensate, and may progress to one of the cardiac arrest rhythms, like ventricular fibrillation. Some very slow rhythms such as third-degree AV block can also be electrically unstable, because cardiac output is relying upon an escape rhythm only, which can stop at any time.

Rhythms that are haemodynamically and/or electrically unstable:

- Rapid, sustained ventricular tachycardia.
- Third degree AV block, or high second degree AV block, where the heart rate is less than 40 beats/minute, or there are pauses between the ventricular escape complexes.
- Atrial standstill as a result of hyperkalaemia.
- Arrest rhythms such as asystole, ventricular fibrillation or pulseless bradyarrhythmias.

TACHYARRHYTHMIAS

ATRIAL FIBRILLATION

This is the most common persistent arrhythmia seen in small animal medicine, and is usually seen as a result of structural heart disease. Rapid and irregular depolarisation occurs across the atria, some of which make it through the AV node. It is not unusual

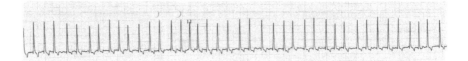

Figure 5.23 Atrial fibrillation. Heart rate is 229 beats/minute.

that the atria may be contracting at a rate over 300 beats/minute, but what is conducted through the AV node may be 200 beats/minute.

ECG CHARACTERISTICS

It is a normal to fast rhythm, and the interval between R waves is irregular. There are no obvious P waves associated with the QRS complexes, and the QRS complexes often vary in amplitude (size). The complexes are tall and narrow, because they have originated in the atria. Figure 5.23 illustrates atrial fibrillation on an ECG trace.

CLINICAL FINDINGS

On auscultation, the heart sounds chaotic and irregular. There is often a marked difference between heart rate and pulse rate, so pulse deficits are a common finding. Atrial fibrillation is usually present with heart failure, so patients often show signs of left sided congestive heart failure and are usually exercise intolerant.

Nursing actions

- Keep patient calm, avoiding stress and give medication for heart failure if present.
- Any exercise should be for toileting purposes only, and done so slowly and gently.

VENTRICULAR TACHYCARDIA

Ventricular tachycardia occurs when three or more ventricular premature complexes occur together, at a sustained rate of 150 beats/minute or more. It is usually associated with severe cardiac disease or systemic disease. It is particularly prevalent in Dobermans and Boxers with cardiomyopathy. It can also be seen secondary to conditions such as splenic mass, electrolyte disturbances or as a consequence of some drugs.

ECG CHARACTERISTICS

This is a fast rhythm, that may or may not be sustained. Complexes are wide and bizarre, and most commonly are uniform in appearance, but can be multiform. P waves are usually not visible because the QRS waves are much bigger. Figure 5.24 shows an example of a ventricular run, amongst an otherwise sinus rhythm.

CLINICAL FINDINGS

Because of the possible dramatic effect ventricular tachycardia can have on cardiac output, rapid ventricular tachycardia can be life threatening if left untreated, because it can develop into ventricular fibrillation and cause sudden death.

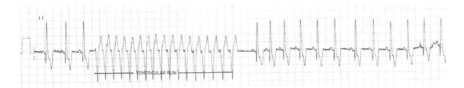

Figure 5.24 Ventricular tachycardia. Note the three sinus complexes, the run of ventricular tachycardia, and the return of sinus rhythm.

Nursing actions

- A veterinary surgeon must be informed immediately.
- An intravenous catheter should be placed and emergency drugs, such as lidocaine, be ready for use.
- An ECG should be attached.
- The patient should be kept calm and handled gently.

BRADYARRHYTHMIAS

ATRIOVENTRICULAR BLOCK

Atrioventricular block occurs when the electrical impulse is not conducted normally through the AV node. There are three classifications of AV block:

First degree AV block

This occurs when conduction is slowed through the AV node. It has the appearance of a sinus rhythm, but the P–R interval is prolonged. It is quite rare, and can be difficult to identify. No abnormalities will be found on auscultation, as it is almost indistinguishable from sinus rhythm.

Second degree AV block

This occurs when conduction fails occasionally. The SA node initiates P waves normally, but some of them fail to be conducted through the AV node, and therefore do not produce a corresponding QRS complex. Second degree AV block can often be seen in veterinary practice, and is caused by increased vagal tone, structural heart disease, or drugs (such as alpha-2 agonists like medetomidine).

ECG characteristics

There are some P-QRS sinus complexes present, but some P waves occur without corresponding QRS complexes. Second degree AV block can be classified further:

Mobitz type I – The P-R interval increases (the distance between the P wave and the QRS complex) before the block. Figure 5.25 is an example of Mobitz type I.

Mobitz type II – The P-R interval remains the same before the block. Often the frequency of the block is constant, for example two sinus complexes for one unconducted P wave, or three to one, etc.

Uncconducted
P waves

Unconducted
P waves

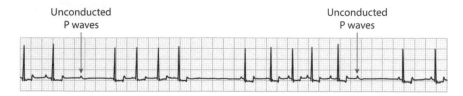

Figure 5.25 Example of 2nd degree AV block. Heart rate is 86 beats/minute. This example is Mobitz type I because the P-R interval changes on the trace. Arrows denote unconducted P waves.

Clinical findings

Depending on the intrinsic heart rate, second degree AV block may or may not be clinically significant. If the heart rate is very slow, haemodynamic compromise can occur, and a patient may present with signs of lethargy, exercise intolerance, or syncope. Sometimes an additional heart sound can be heard (S4) which is associated with atrial depolarisation.

Nursing actions

- Consider if there is clinical significance, by assessing the patient and what is happening to it at that time. If there is cardiac compromise, inform a veterinary surgeon immediately.
- If the block is anaesthesia or sedation related, consider reducing the volatile agent, or reversing the alpha-2 agonist.
- Monitor heart rate and blood pressure.

Third degree AV block

Third degree AV block (also known as complete AV block) is seen when no P waves are conducted through the AV node at all. It occurs when there is a persistent failure of conduction. It is an electrically unstable rhythm and may need urgent veterinary attention because the escape mechanism can fail. Cats generally have a higher ventricular escape rate (approximately 100 beats/minute or more), therefore, clinical signs are less severe.

ECG characteristics

The ECG shows regular P waves, with a slower and spontaneous ventricular or junctional (AV node) rhythm, independent of the P waves. These wide and bizarre complexes are essential to maintain cardiac output, and are often referred to as escape complexes. Figure 5.26 shows an example of third degree AV block in a dog, and 5.27 shows a cat trace.

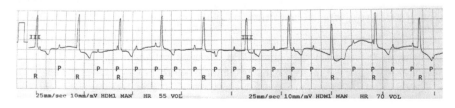

Figure 5.26 Example of third degree AV block in a dog.

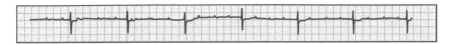

Figure 5.27 Example of third degree AV block in a cat. Heart rate is 40 beats/minute. Note that the atrial rate is significantly different to the ventricular, or escape rate.

Clinical findings

Patients that present in third degree AV block can have clinical signs such as syncope, weakness or even sudden death. Once potential causes such as neoplasia have been ruled out, pacemaker implantation may be considered. An S4 additional heart sound may be heard in some cases.

Nursing actions

- If cardiac output is compromised, inform a veterinary surgeon immediately.
- Treat patient symptomatically, avoiding stress and exertion.

ATRIAL STANDSTILL

As the name suggests, there is no atrial activity with this rhythm, and it is usually a slow rhythm. It is often seen with hyperkalaemia. Figure 5.28 shows atrial standstill.

ECG characteristics

Absence of P waves and escape complexes may be ventricular or junctional.

Clinical findings

Normal heart sounds are present with atrial standstill, but at a slower rate than normal. Clinical signs include syncope, lethargy, and weakness.

Nursing actions

- If cardiac output is compromised, inform a veterinary surgeon immediately.
- Blood sample may be needed to confirm diagnosis.
- IV catheter equipment and fluids or calcium to be used as necessary.
- Treat patient as prescribed by the veterinary surgeon, avoiding stress and exertion.

ARREST RHYTHMS

There are three main arrest rhythms that can be identified on ECG.

- *Ventricular fibrillation* – Originating from multiple foci in the ventricles, it produces very little cardiac output. The reasons for ventricular fibrillation can be numerous and the underlying medical condition needs to be known. An example of this is seen in Figure 5.29.

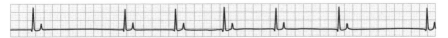

Figure 5.28 Atrial standstill. Heart rate is 40 beats/minute. Note the complete lack of P waves. This was a patient diagnosed with Addisons disease.

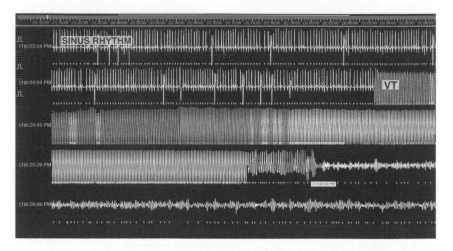

Figure 5.29 Progression of an arrhythmia to ventricular fibrillation. The trace starts with sinus rhythm with occasional VPCs, progresses to ventricular tachycardia and ultimately ventricular fibrillation. Note in ventricular fibrillation there is no coordinated ventricular contraction. VPC = Ventricular premature complex. VT = Ventricular tachycardia. VF = Ventricular fibrillation.

- *Ventricular standstill* – P waves may be visible, but no QRS activity. No discernible pulse.
- *Pulseless electrical activity* – QRS complexes are visible on the ECG trace, but no discernible pulse is felt at the same time. It is usually a slow rhythm and may occur with severe acidosis, hypoxaemia, and hyperkalaemia.

Nursing actions

- Attract attention immediately for assistance and inform a veterinary surgeon.
- Cardiopulmonary resuscitation (CPR) started straight away.

KEY POINTS

- Stop! What is the patient telling you?
- Is the patient collapsed? Get a veterinary surgeon immediately.
- Is the patient weak? Get a veterinary surgeon immediately.
- Is the patient standing and alert? Avoid stress and inform the veterinary surgeon.
- What is the heart rate? It is what you would expect for the species, breed, and age?
- What are the pulses like? Is it strong, weak or irregular? Are there pulse deficits?
- Is blood pressure lower than expected?
- Can the anaesthetic be decreased?
- If unsure, speak to a veterinary surgeon.

FURTHER READING

Fletcher DJ, Boller M, Brainard BM, Steven CH et al. (2012). RECOVER evidence and knowledge gap analysis on veterinary CPR. Part 7: Clinical guidelines. *Journal of Veterinary Emergency and Critical Care.* 22 (Suppl 1):S102–31. https://doi.org/10.1111/j.1476-4431.2012.00757.x.

Martin M (2015). *Small Animal ECGs: An Introductory Guide.* 3rd edition, Wiley Blackwell, Oxford.

6

The nurse's role in diagnostic tests

Patients with cardiac disease will need diagnostic tests, either as part of a screening programme, to confirm a diagnosis, monitor disease progression, or assess efficacy of treatment. This chapter looks at how the nurse can be prepared for tests, produce reliable and repeatable results, whilst minimising stress to the patient.

AUSCULTATION

Auscultation is used to listen to the heart rate and rhythm, and the heart and lung sounds. There are two normal heart sounds in the dog and cat, the 'lub' and 'dub'. The 'lub' sound is the atrioventricular valves closing, and is known as S1. The 'dub' sound is known as S2, and is heard when the semilunar valves close. S1 is a louder, longer, and duller sound than S2. S2 is a shorter higher pitched sound. Any other sounds are described as additional heart sounds. Box 6.1 summarises the heart sounds. These extra sounds are described by location, or the point of maximal intensity (PMI), by the timing in the cardiac cycle, and intensity of the sound (loudness).

THE STETHOSCOPE

Figure 6.1 shows the main components of a stethoscope. The binaurals should face forward and fit snugly into the ears. It may be necessary to move the tubing up or down to better fit the ear canal and minimise sound leakage. The diaphragm is used to hear high pitched sounds in the lungs and heart, and is best for hearing heart sounds S1 and S2. The bell is used for lower pitched heart sounds and extra heart sounds. Some stethoscopes do not have a separate bell and diaphragm, so fingertip pressure can be used to distinguish between high and low-pitched sounds.

BOX 6.1: Heart sounds

S1   Lub. Atrioventricular valves closing. A longer, louder, and duller sound. Occurs with a pulse.

S2 – Dub. Semilunar valves closing. A shorter higher pitched sound. Occurs after the pulse.

S3 and S4 sounds occur in diastole are called gallop sounds because they sound like a galloping horse. It is very difficult to distinguish between S3 and S4 sounds.

DOI: 10.1201/9781003122173-7

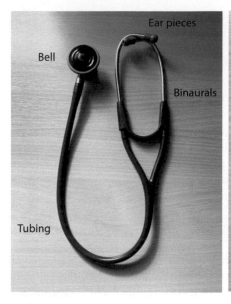
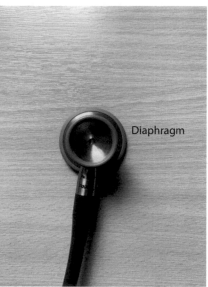

Figure 6.1 Picture of stethoscope labelled.

AUSCULTATION TECHNIQUE

A good technique is needed to maximise auscultation. Common artefacts that can hamper auscultation include shaking, movement, panting, purring, and increased respiratory noise. Try to calm the patient as much as possible to create optimal listening conditions. Below is a guide to good technique. Table 6.1 summarizes auscultation techniques for each heart valve.

- The patient should be in a standing position, in a quiet room.
- Both sides of the entire thorax should be auscultated. The heart should be auscultated separately from the lungs.
- Listen to the heart rate and rhythm, and note if the respiratory pattern changes it (such as respiratory mediated sinus arrhythmia).
- Take time to recognise normal heart sounds, the lub and dub. If extra heart sounds are identified, the next steps are to localise and identify the PMI, timing, and intensity.
- All valve areas should be auscultated in order, starting with the pulmonic valve moving to the aortic, mitral, and then tricuspid valves.
- Starting with the left side of the thorax, move the stethoscope from base to apex, starting with the pulmonic area. It may be necessary to move the left leg forward so that the third intercostal space, the site of the pulmonic valve, can be heard better.
- Move slightly upwards and back one intercostal space to maximise the area of the aortic valve. It may not be possible to distinguish the aortic and pulmonic areas in small dogs and cats. This is the case in Figure 6.2.
- The sternum in cats should also be auscultated, as seen in Figure 6.3.

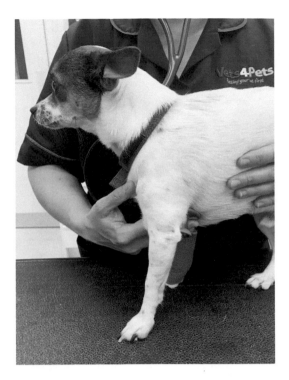

Figure 6.2 Auscultation of the heart base for the pulmonic and aortic valves, on the left hand side of the thorax.

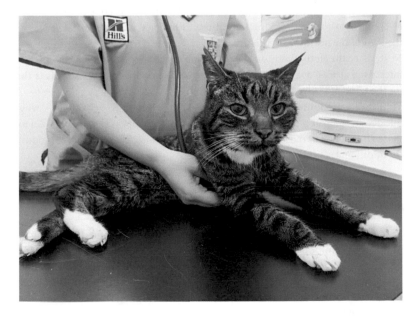

Figure 6.3 Auscultation of the sternum in cats.

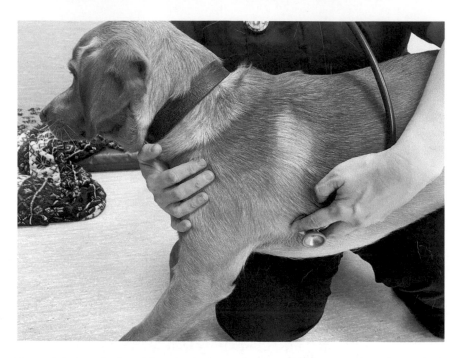

Figure 6.4 Auscultation of the mitral valve, at the apex of the heart on the right hand side of the thorax.

- Remaining on the left side of the thorax, move the stethoscope a little lower to the level of the costochondral junctions at the fifth to seventh intercostal spaces. This is the PMI of the mitral valve (Figure 6.4).
- Next, place the stethoscope on the right side of the thorax between the third to fifth intercostal spaces, again at the level of the costochondral junctions. This is the PMI for the tricuspid valve (Figure 6.5).
- Timing of any additional heart sounds needs to be noted. To help identify when systole occurs, palpate a pulse at the same time as auscultation (Figure 6.6). An arterial pulse should be felt during systole, between S1 and S2. The intensity, or loudness of the additional sounds should be noted.

TIMING OF ADDITIONAL HEART SOUNDS

Additional heart sounds that are heard between S1 and S2 are occurring during systole. This is the most common type of heart murmur in small animals. Sounds heard between S2 and S1 are diastolic murmurs. Diastolic murmurs are rare in small animal medicine. Murmurs that are heard throughout systole and diastole are called continuous murmurs. Figure 6.7 shows a phonocardiograph trace illustrating when a systolic murmur can be heard in the cardiac cycle.

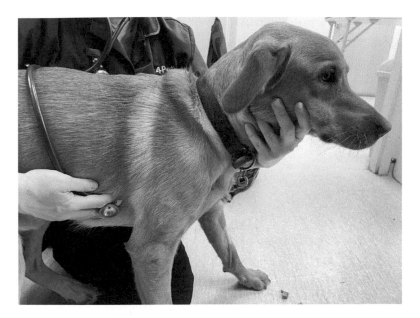

Figure 6.5 Auscultation of the tricuspid valve, at the apex of the heart on the right hand side of the thorax.

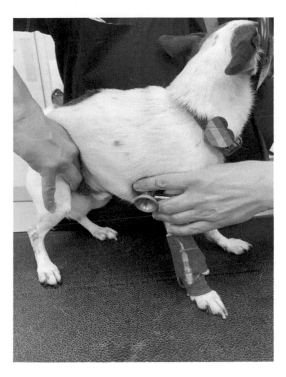

Figure 6.6 Auscultation whilst palpating pulses, such as the femoral artery, can help identify pulse deficits.

Table 6.1 Summary to maximise auscultation technique

Structure	Location
Mitral valve (left apex)	Dog – left side, 5th intercostal space at costochondral junction.
	Cat – Left side, 5th–6th intercostal space, near sternum.
Aortic valve (left base)	Dog – Left side, 4th intercostal just above costochondral junction.
	Cat – left side 2nd–3rd intercostal space just dorsal to pulmonic area.
Pulmonic valve (left base)	Dog – Left side, between 2nd and 4th intercostal space, just above sternum.
	Cat – Left side, 2nd–3rd intercostal space, one third of the way up from sternum.
Tricuspid valve (right apex)	Dog – Right side, 3rd–5th intercostal space near costochondral junction.
	Cat – Right side, 4th–5th intercostal space near sternum.

HEART MURMURS

A heart murmur is classified as any abnormal heart sound of prolonged duration. It can occur because blood is flowing through an abnormal valve (seen with myxomatous mitral valve disease, Chapter 2), due to the narrowing of a vessel (either aortic or pulmonic stenosis, Chapter 4), or because the heart has to work faster to handle more blood quicker than normal. Heart murmurs can occur when there is no heart disease present. For example, innocent or physiological murmurs can be quite normal for puppies and kittens that disappear by the age of six months. These murmurs are usually left sided and are low grade (less than III/VI). Innocent murmurs can still be present in adult cats and dogs, but if no disease is suspected, no treatment is required.

Heart murmurs may also be heard in patients with severe anaemia, which is caused by low viscosity of the blood. When the anaemia is corrected, the murmur can disappear. Table 6.2 summarises possible causes of heart murmurs.

GRADING OF HEART MURMURS

The loudness, or intensity of heart sounds are recorded according to a grading system.

Grade I – A low intensity murmur, heard only in quiet environment after careful auscultation. Quieter than other heart sounds.

Grade II – A low intensity murmur heard immediately when stethoscope is placed over the PMI. Approximately as loud as the other heart sounds.

Grade III – A murmur of moderate intensity. Clearly louder than the other heart sounds.

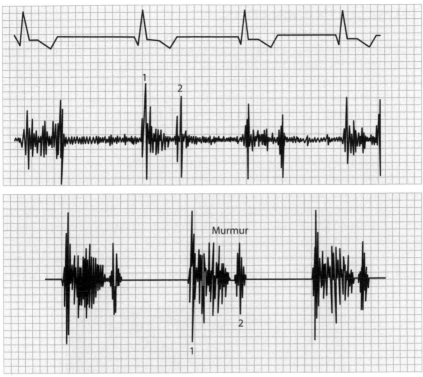

Line 1 - ECG trace to show timings of heart sounds
Line 2 - Phonocardiograph recording showing where heart sounds are situated in relation to the ECG trace.
Line 3 - Indicates when a systolic heart murmur can be heard

Figure 6.7 Diagram showing when a systolic heart murmur sound can be heard in the cardiac cycle.

Grade IV – High intensity murmur that can be heard over several areas.

Grade V – High intensity with a palpable precordial thrill. To the observer, a thrill feels like a syringe of water being pushed against the fingers.

Grade VI – High intensity murmur with a palpable precordial thrill, that may be heard when the stethoscope is slightly lifted off the chest.

Table 6.2 Causes of heart murmurs

Heart disease	Flow murmurs	Other causes
Leaking valves (e.g., mitral valve disease)	Innocent murmurs	Anaemia
Stenotic valves (e.g., pulmonic stenosis)	Physiological murmurs	Hyperthyroidism
Holes in the heart (e.g., ventricular septal defects)		
Abnormal communication between vessels (e.g., patent ductus arteriosus)		

PHYSICAL EXAMINATION

Physical examination is an important part of assessment and should be done without causing stress to the patient. Without even touching the patient, much information can be gathered, such as respiratory rate, pattern, and effort. Some patients may present in respiratory distress, and in some, audible pulmonary crackles can be heard without a stethoscope. Some patients that have been diagnosed with chronic heart failure, may present with paradoxical breathing. Any patient that presents with increased respiratory rate or effort should be handled cautiously, minimising stress, and keeping as calm as possible. This may mean hospitalising the patient away from other dogs or cats.

Body and muscle condition scoring can also occur without handling the patient. A patient with ascites will have a distended pendulous abdomen, and will likely be unable to get comfortable. A patient with cardiac cachexia may have muscle wastage, especially from the temporal head muscles (Figure 6.8), poor coat condition, prominent ribs, and spine. Figure 6.9 shows an example of cardiac cachexia.

Heart rate and rhythm can be assessed as described above. Pulse rate and quality are useful, especially when combined with auscultation (Figure 6.6), as this may help with

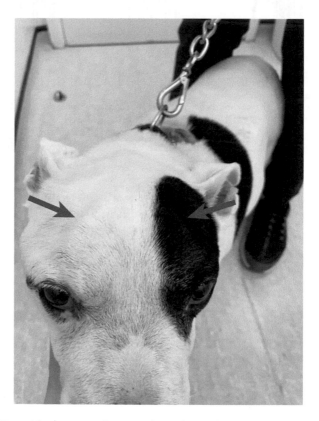

Figure 6.8 Dog with pronounced temporal muscle wastage.

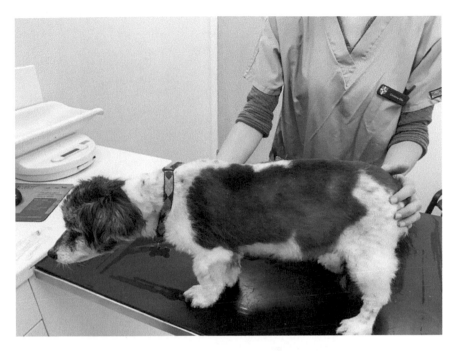

Figure 6.9 Dog with cardiac cachexia. It has a prominent spine and poor coat condition.

working out timing of heart murmurs in the cardiac cycle, or detect pulse deficits, which are found with arrhythmias. Patients that are collapsed may have weak or absent pulses, and cold extremities. Box 6.2 summarises pulse quality assessment.

Assessing mucous membrane colour can be useful, if it does not stress the patient (Box 6.3). If a patient is cyanotic or grey as a result of hypoxia, significant oxygen deprivation

BOX 6.2: Assessing pulse quality

Weak/thready pulses – poor circulation
Fast or irregular pulses – Possibly as a result of an arrhythmia
Water hammer pulses – Strong, jerky pulse quality. Found with patent ductus arteriosus.

BOX 6.3: Mucous membrane colour seen in cardiac patients

Pink – Normal
Pallor – Pale. Result of forward heart failure or anaemia. Capillary refill time may be delayed.
Cyanosis or grey – Hypoxia. Result of congestive heart failure.

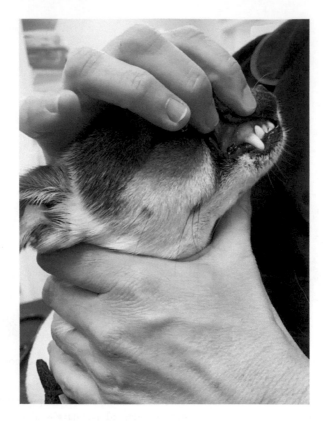

Figure 6.10 Example of normal mucous membrane colour.

has already occurred, and the patient should be handled minimally, and placed in an oxygen rich environment. Figure 6.10 shows normal mucous membrane colour.

Temperature taking can be problematic. If a patient is stressed by the process, it should not be done, and the question raised as to why it is necessary. However, recording a temperature can provide valuable information for a cat presenting with an aortic thromboembolism, as lower rectal temperatures are associated with poorer prognosis. If a patient is receiving oxygen therapy in a confined environment, it may be desirable to ensure that the patient is not overheating.

BLOOD PRESSURE

Blood pressure is used to assess cardiac output, rule out concurrent diseases like hypertension and renal disease, and monitor treatment. Non-invasive blood pressure is best done in a reliable and repeatable method, with notes made on the file, so that the conditions can be reproduced on the next assessment. The Doppler method, if available, is the preferred approach, although oscillometric may benefit patients that cannot tolerate

BOX 6.4: Blood pressure equipment list

An assistant or owner for restraint, if necessary. Remember, less is often more with
  scared patients.
Doppler ultrasound machine and sphygmomanometer, or oscillometric device
Ultrasound gel
Appropriate size cuff, pre-tested
Tape to secure cuff if needed
Swab pre-soaked with surgical spirit OR clippers
Headphones if desired
Paper to record results
Pen

being restrained for any period of time. Advances in blood pressure monitoring means
that high definition oscillometry machines are now available, and have been shown to be
as reliable as Doppler. What is important is that whatever method is used, it is repeated so
that an accurate trend can be reported.

How to take blood pressure

- Plan how the test will be performed, before handling the patient. Use a quite kennel
  or room. Prepare the equipment (Box 6.4), ensuring that the volume is turned off on
  the machine, or use headphones
- Select an appropriate cuff before starting and test it to ensure it holds inflation.
- If measuring blood pressure in a cat, and performing the test in a different room and
  not in a kennel, allow 5–10 minutes for the cat to acclimatise to the new surround-
  ings. If the cat is more comfortable in its basket, allow it to remain in it. If this is not
  possible, remove the cat from the basket and allow it to sit as comfortably as possible
  and restrain gently.
- Place the cuff gently, but securely, around the chosen area (radial or coccygeal artery).
  If tape is used to secure the cuff, do not encompass the whole cuff, as this will restrict
  the cuff's ability to inflate.
- It is not always necessary to clip the area, so try without, if the patient is scared. Wipe
  the area with a surgical spirit soaked swab. If clippers are used, clip the site in one
  movement, to minimise stress.
- If headphones are used, place on head and test the sound. Use as little sound as possible.
- Apply ultrasound gel to the Doppler probe and confidently but gently place on the
  artery to be tested.
- Increase the volume and inflate the cuff to approximately 20 mmHg above where the
  Doppler signal is lost. Wherever the blood pressure is being taken, the Doppler probe
  should be at the approximate level of the right atrium.
- Deflate the cuff slowly but completely and note when the systolic 'whoosh' sound is
  clearly audible. Repeat up to six times in total, discarding the first reading. It is also
  good practice to take a pulse rate at the same time. Record all numbers and work out
  an average.

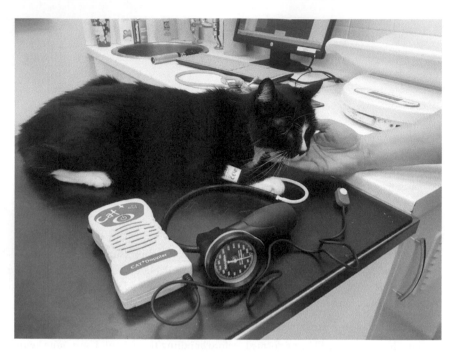

Figure 6.11 Equipment prepared and ready for use in cat.

- Once the measurements have been taken, turn off the Doppler machine, wipe the gel from the patient, remove the cuff, and return to its kennel, basket or owner.
- It is also useful to record the demeanour of the patient (such as excited, calm, dull) when the test was performed, as this could vary results.
- Figure 6.11 shows blood pressure equipment ready for use in a cat; Figure 6.12 shows blood pressure in a dog; Figure 6.13 shows stress-free blood pressure measurement in a cat; and Figure 6.14 shows stress-free blood pressure measurement in a dog.

If an oscillometric machine is used to measure blood pressure, use the technique described above and record systolic, diastolic, and mean pressures.

BLOOD SAMPLING

Blood sampling is often required in cardiac patients. It may be needed to rule out concurrent diseases, such as anaemia, hyperthyroidism, or renal disease, or it may be required to establish a baseline on renal and electrolyte parameters before diuresis is started. If blood sampling is required in cardiac patients, stress should be minimised, especially if the patient is in heart failure. These are not patients to be practiced on, so experienced or trained veterinary professionals should be the ones taking the samples. Sampling should be achieved by working with the patient, which may not conform to normal sampling

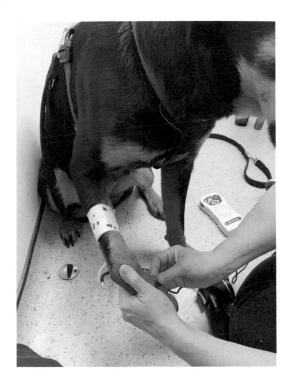

Figure 6.12 Placement of ultrasound probe on a dog. Note that the paw is raised to the level of right atrium.

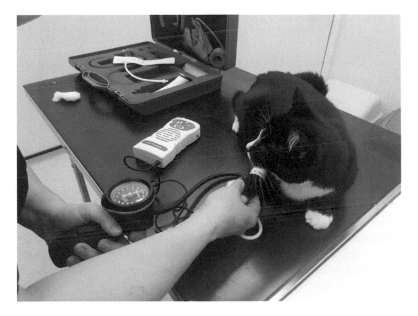

Figure 6.13 Blood pressure in a cat.

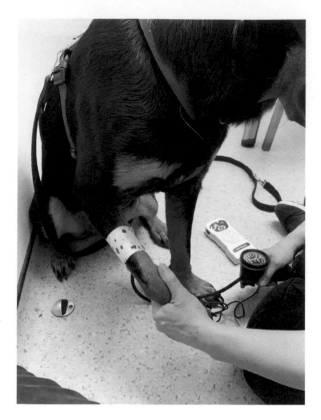

Figure 6.14 Blood pressure in a dog. Both the cat and dog blood pressure measurements were taken in the consult room so the patient did not have to see other dogs or cats.

conventions. Venepuncture tips are shown in Figure 6.15. Examples of blood sampling techniques are shown in Figures 6.16 and 6.17.

RADIOGRAPHY

Thoracic radiography can provide useful diagnostic information to rule out other disease processes, such as lung disease or neoplasia. In dogs with heart disease, chamber enlargement can be identified, especially if it used as part of a series, charting disease progression. It is also helpful to diagnose if heart failure is present, and assess the efficacy of diuresis in dogs. It is limited however, because it is not sensitive for mild to moderate forms of heart disease, and the pattern of pulmonary oedema in cats is variable. Further, for both cats and dogs, the benefits that may be gained need to outweigh the safety of taking radiographs, whether that be lying in lateral recumbency when presenting with heart failure, or the risk of sedation.

Positioning is very important, so that all of the lung fields can be visualised. If more than one view is required, the dorsoventral (DV) view should be taken first, and lateral views

Take the sample in a quiet area, preferably where a door can be locked to prevent disruption.

Often, less is more with cardiac patients. Try using minimal restraint when blood sampling.

Only a competent holder and venepuncturist should take samples on stressed patients.

If some blood has been obtained, consider how little is actually needed.

Give the patient time to rest between attempts.

Dogs

Consider using alternative veins. If haematology is not needed, a lateral saphenous vein can be used with the dog standing and made a fuss of at the front. It is often tolerated well.

Sampling with the patient on the floor may decrease stress.

Use distraction to allow sampling to occur. A slightly open door can be really helpful, as long as someone has the dog on a lead, so it cannot escape.

Consider taking blood with the owner present, if that calms the dog.

Cats

A towel wrapped securely but not tightly around a cat's body can provide security and prevent feet protruding.

A cat friendly veterinary professional is ideal for sampling and restraint.

Scruffing is not acceptable practice.

Figure 6.15 Tips to stress free venepuncture.

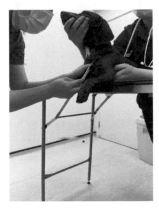

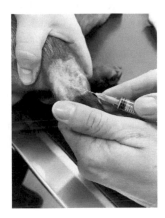

Figure 6.16 Photograph of jugular blood sampling.

Figure 6.17 Photograph of sampling a lateral saphenous vein.

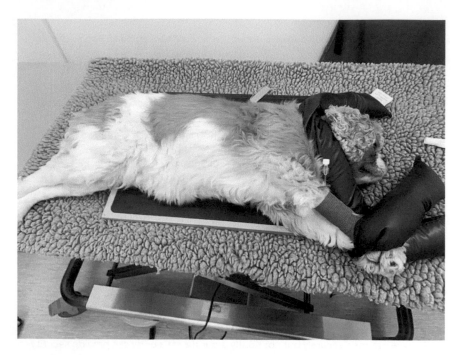

Figure 6.18 Positioning for lateral thoracic radiographs.

subsequently, so that the lungs are not compromised on the first view. Ideally, radiographs should be taken on inspiration, but if the patient is breathing rapidly or panting, it may be preferable to take the radiograph on expiration to minimise movement blur. The images may not be perfect, but for the purposes of assessing whether heart failure is present, they may be sufficient. Optimal positioning for thoracic radiography is seen in Figure 6.18 and 6.19. Figures 6.20 and 6.21 show DV and lateral thorax canine radiographs of a healthy dog. Figures 6.22 and 6.23 show lateral and DV radiographs of a dog in severe heart failure. Note the size of the cardiac silhouette and whiteness of the lungs, compared to Figures 6.20 and 6.21.

How to achieve good quality thoracic radiographs:

- Have the X-ray machine ready with settings, patient details in the processor, and views selected.
- Have an oxygen supply ready, with a mask, or just a circuit, if a mask is not tolerated.
- Two views are preferred – DV and a right lateral. Take the DV view first if possible, but work to what the patient can tolerate
- Use high kV, low mAs.
- Good positioning is important. Try to minimise thoracic rotation, and pull the fore-limbs forward.
- Take at peak inspiration, unless panting or tachypnoeic.

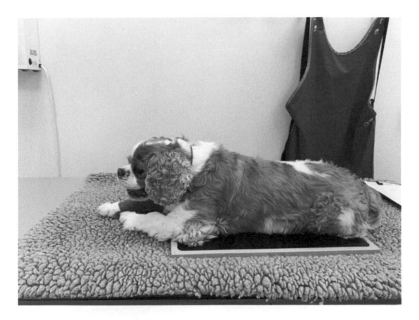

Figure 6.19 Positioning for DV thoracic radiographs. A sandbag was added across the neck at the last minute to minimise stress.

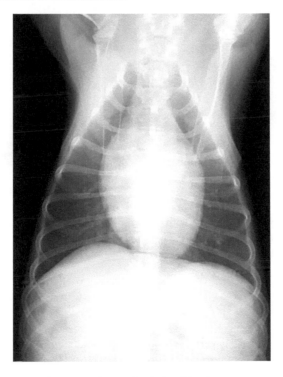

Figure 6.20 Canine DV thoracic radiograph of a healthy dog.

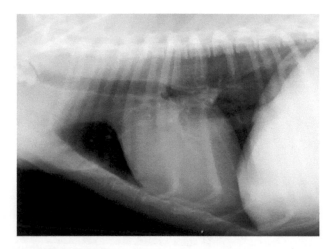

Figure 6.21 Canine lateral thoracic radiograph of a healthy dog.

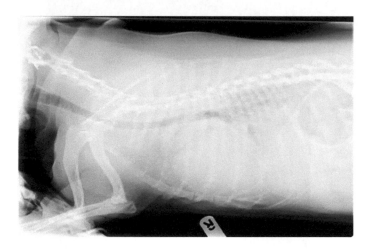

Figure 6.22 Canine lateral thoracic radiograph of a dog with severe heart failure.

Always handle dyspnoeic patients with care, allow rest periods and provide supplemental oxygen, if tolerated. Nurses have a crucial role in assessing whether a patient is fit for radiography, and should raise any concerns to the veterinary surgeon.

ECHOCARDIOGRAPHY

Nurses may not necessarily perform echocardiography, but they can be integral in preparing the patient and monitoring it whilst the scan is happening. As with all diagnostic tests, stress should be minimised, and if possible, should be performed in a quiet room

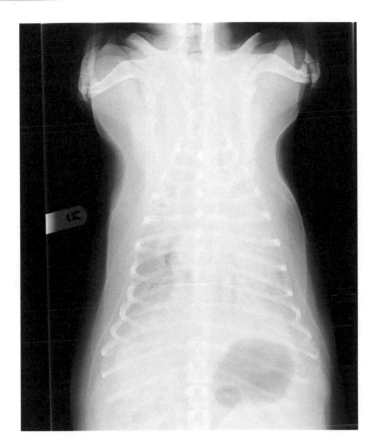

Figure 6.23 Canine DV thoracic radiograph of a dog with severe heart failure.

with minimal distractions. Echocardiography is the gold standard diagnostic test for heart disease diagnosis. It is however, a difficult skill to master, and so, if no cardiologist is available, or the patient is unstable, a 'focused point-of-care' exam, or lung ultrasound at the kennel, can assess for abnormal fluid accumulation, such as pulmonary oedema, pleural or pericardial effusions. It can also be used to estimate left atrial size and left ventricular (LV) systolic function.

The following should act as a guide for preparation:

- Have the ultrasound machine on and ready for the individual patient.
- Ensure enough ultrasound gel in the bottle and placed next to the machine.
- Have paper towel and/or tongue depressor nearby to clean the patient when the scan has finished.
- Place surgical spirit next to machine.
- Prepare a comfortable bed for patient to lie on.
- Ensure clippers are available and work. Try to use quiet clippers if possible.

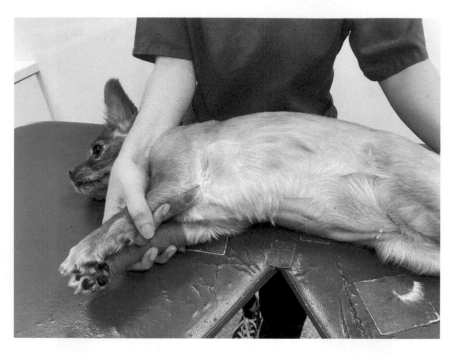

Figure 6.24 Patient prepared for echocardiography, lying in right lateral recumbency. Note the clip patch at the cranial thorax behind the left forelimb. This same area has been clipped on the right lateral side also. A small window has also been clipped on the ventral abdomen at the xiphisternum. This allows aortic velocities (pressure of blood flow through the aorta) to be measured.

- Clip patient on both sides of the thorax (Figure 6.24). As an easy rule, feel where the heartbeat is, clip that spot and cranially towards the axilla.
- When the veterinary surgeon is ready, place the patient in lateral recumbency. Right lateral is usually preferred to start.
- If the patient is dyspnoeic, a scan can be performed in sternal recumbency if it is a cat, or standing if a dog. Alternatively, a point of care thoracic ultrasound can be performed instead.

During the scan, monitor the patient closely. If they have been or are currently in heart failure, monitor respiratory rate and effort. Supplementary oxygen may be necessary, but should not stress the patient. If the patient becomes stressed, allow breaks for the patient to rest.

Ideally, sedation is not recommended for echocardiography because cardiac parameters can be affected. It is paramount therefore, that the nurse monitors the environment and observes the patient closely.

KEY POINTS

- Diagnostic tests are a valuable part of diagnosis and monitoring in cardiac patients.
- Nurses have a crucial role in ensuring tests are reliable and repeatable, that stress is minimised, and that patient welfare comes before any diagnostic test.
- Echocardiography is the most useful diagnostic test for heart disease, because it can provide information on chamber size and function, assess blood flow patterns, and allow visualisation of spontaneous echo contrast or thrombi (Chapter 3).

FURTHER READING

Acierno MJ, Brown S, Coleman AE, Jepson RE, Papich M, Stepien RL, Syme HM (2018). ACVIM consensus statement: Guidelines for the identification, evaluation, and management of systemic hypertension in dogs and cats. *Journal of Veterinary Internal Medicine*. 32(6):1803–1822.

7

Drugs

This chapter will look at the drugs most commonly used in treating heart disease and heart failure in dogs and cats. Most drugs are used at the onset of clinical signs, but recent advances in veterinary canine cardiac pharmacology mean that treatment can now be used to slow the progression from moderate disease to heart failure. A brief section on antiarrhythmic treatment is also included.

The aim of drug therapy in chronic heart failure is to control clinical signs, allowing as good a quality of life for the patient, for as long as possible. The aim of drug therapy in acute life-threatening heart failure is to prevent certain death from respiratory compromise or cardiogenic shock.

There are three target areas that cardiac pharmacology focuses on

1. *Natriuresis and diuresis* – Promoting sodium and water excretion via the kidneys.
2. *Contraction and relaxation of the myocardium* – Improving the pumping action of the heart.
3. Antagonising the deleterious neurohormonal messengers that are activated in heart failure.

NATRIURESIS AND DIURESIS

Diuretics are the first line drug in the treatment of heart failure, and act by removing excess fluid by increasing urine output. There are different groups of diuretics that act on different parts of the kidney. Figure 7.1 indicates where the different groups act, and Table 7.1 summarises the groups and drug doses.

FUROSEMIDE

The most commonly used diuretic is furosemide, a potent drug that works on the loop of Henle, and blocks the absorption of sodium, chloride, and water. Diuretics are indicated for use in most cases with congestive heart failure (CHF). Doses are usually titrated to the minimum effective dose allowing room to manoeuvre upwards when more is needed. There is no evidence to prove the efficacy of furosemide, but it is considered irreplaceable in the treatment of CHF. In some cases, thoracocentesis or pericardiocentesis may be recommended instead of, or in addition to, standard diuretic therapy.

TORASEMIDE

This is a newer loop diuretic. It is more potent and has longer bioavailability than furosemide. It is useful to add to the treatment regime if and when a patient becomes refractory

DOI: 10.1201/9781003122173-8

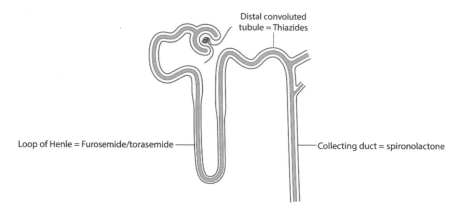

Figure 7.1 Diagram of kidney nephron showing the where different diuretics act.

to furosemide. In addition, at a time when the number of medications can increase, it is only administered once a day.

SPIRONOLACTONE

A potassium sparing diuretic that works on the collecting duct. Spironolactone also has aldosterone agonist properties, and therefore is also used for neurohormonal blockade.

THIAZIDES

Thiazides like hydrochlorothiazide, work on the distal convoluted tubule. They are usually prescribed at the refractory stage of CHF. However, since the introduction of torasemide, it is rarely used.

ADVERSE EFFECTS OF DIURESIS

Polyuria, polydipsia, hypokalaemia, increased urea and creatinine, continuous activation of the renin-angiotensin-aldosterone system (RAAS).

Table 7.1 Summary of diuretics

Class	Location of action	Example	Form	Dose
Loop	Loop of Henle	Furosemide	Injection for IV or IM use, tablet, oral solution	1–6 mg/kg q1–24 h. Titrated to lowest dose possible.
		Torasemide	Tablet	0.1–0.6 mg/kg q24 h
Thiazides	Distal convoluted tubule	Hydrochlorothiazide	Tablet	0.5–2 mg/kg
Potassium sparing	Collecting duct	Spironolcatone	Tablet	1–2 mg/kg q12–24 h

RECOMMENDED NURSING ACTIONS

- *In chronic cases of CHF* – Allow patients access to urinate regularly.
- *In acute cases of CHF* – Check bedding frequently. Minimise stress by having clean bedding ready, and have someone help calm the patient as it is changed.
- Water must always be available.
- Regular blood tests should monitor renal and electrolyte parameters to avoid over diuresis.
- In patients receiving sequential nephron blockade, blood pressure should also be monitored regularly to avoid compromising cardiac output.

CONTRACTION AND RELAXATION OF THE MYOCARDIUM

Another group of drugs used in the management of heart disease are positive inotropes. They help the pumping action of the heart, by increasing contractility of the myocardium. Table 7.2 summarises the positive inotropes class and doses.

PIMOBENDAN

Pimobendan is the most commonly used positive inotrope. Recent developments have meant that it is licensed for use in dogs before heart failure occurs. It has been shown to prolong the time to clinical signs of heart failure in the pre-clinical stage of dilated cardiomyopathy (DCM)[1], and at stage B2 of myxomatous mitral valve disease (MMVD)[2]. Pimobendan also has vasodilatory effects which counteracts RAAS activation. Description of these diseases is in Chapter 2.

DIGOXIN

Digoxin is a weak positive inotrope compared to pimobendan and is more commonly used to treat supraventricular arrhythmias like atrial fibrillation, as it decreases heart rate allowing for an improvement in cardiac filling.

ADVERSE EFFECTS OF POSITIVE INOTROPES

Pimobendan is generally well tolerated and is licensed for use in dogs. It is not licensed for use in cats, but cardiologists do prescribe it for some feline cases. It should not be used in cats with outflow tract obstruction.

Table 7.2 Summary of positive inotropes and doses

Drug	Formulation	Dose
Pimobendan	Injection (outside US) or tablet	0.25–0.3 mg/kg q12
Digoxin	Tablet	3–5 micrograms/kg, q12 h

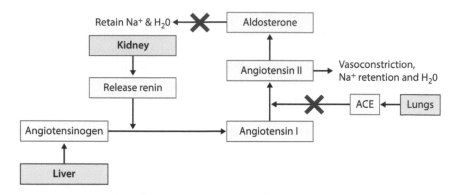

Figure 7.2 Diagram showing where neurohormonal drugs work in the renin-angiotensin-aldosterone system.

Digoxin has a narrow therapeutic window. Adverse effects include gastrointestinal symptoms, bradyarrhythmias and tachyarrhythmias. Blood digoxin levels should be monitored regularly.

RECOMMENDED NURSING ACTIONS

Pimobendan should be administered an hour before feeding to maximize bioavailability.

NEUROHORMONAL BLOCKADE

The purpose of neurohormonal blockade is to antagonise the deleterious neurohormonal messengers that are activated in heart failure. Figure 7.2 shows where the neurohormonal blockers work. Table 7.3 summarises the neurohormonal blocker class and doses.

ANGIOTENSIN CONVERTING ENZYME (ACE) INHIBITORS

Angiotensin converting enzyme (ACE) inhibitors block the neurohormonal conversion of angiotensin I to angiotensin II. Angiotensin II is a hormone produced in heart failure that instigates vasoconstriction and sodium and water retention. An ACE inhibitor therefore, vasodilates blood vessels, and prevents the neurohormonal messages to retain sodium. This means that ACE inhibitors are indicated in most cases where furosemide is prescribed. Examples of ACE inhibitors are enalapril, benazepril, and ramipril. Due to its vasodilatory properties, ACE inhibitors are also used in cases with hypertension.

Table 7.3 Summary of neurohormonal blockers and doses

Drug	Formulation	Dose
Enalapril	Tablet	0.5 mg/kg q12–24 h
Benazepril	Tablet – Licensed for use in cats	0.5–1.0 mg/kg q24 h
Spironolactone	Tablet	1–2 mg/kg q12–24 h

ALDOSTERONE ANTAGONISTS

Aldosterone is another hormone produced in heart failure (see Figure 7.2). It has similar vasoconstriction and sodium retention effects as angiotensin II. An example of an aldosterone antagonist is spironolactone, which is also used for its potassium sparing diuretic properties.

ADVERSE EFFECTS OF NEUROHORMONAL BLOCKADE

Azotaemia and hypotension

RECOMMENDED NURSING ACTIONS

Renal and electrolytes and blood pressure should be monitored regularly.

TREATMENT OF FELINE HEART DISEASE, THROMBOEMBOLISM, AND HEART FAILURE

There is little empirical evidence supporting the treatment of feline cardiac disease, but there are significant differences to the management of canine heart disease. The most striking is that feline heart disease can lead to thrombotic events, that may affect the forelimbs, hindlimbs, or to organs such as the brain, mesentery or kidneys. There are two groups of antithrombotic therapy: antiplatelet drugs and anticoagulant therapy.

- Antiplatelet drugs inhibit some platelet function. Examples are aspirin and clopidogrel.
- Anticoagulants inhibit parts of the coagulation cascade. Examples are warfarin, heparin and rivaroxaban.

Clopidogrel has been shown to be the superior antiplatelet drug for cats[3]. It is recommended in cats that have moderate to large left atrial enlargement but no clinical signs of heart failure (stage B2), or those that have clinical signs of heart failure with moderate to large left atrial enlargement, (stage C). It is also recommended that when a cat has had a thrombotic event, it is given as soon as the cat is able to tolerate oral medication. Box 7.1 summarises the protocol to follow when a cat presents after a thrombotic event.

The American College of Veterinary Internal Medicine consensus statement recommended the following treatment guidelines for feline heart failure[4] (Table 7.4).

RECOMMENDED NURSING ACTIONS

- The cat's welfare needs to be considered before adding multiple medications.
- The cat's welfare also needs to be taken into account when considering re-examination. Owner reports of sleeping respiratory rate can be sufficient in monitoring response to diuresis.

> ## BOX 7.1: Treatment when a cat has presented with a thrombus
>
> - Analgesia is the main priority when a cat presents with an aortic thromboembolism (ATE). It is recommended to use either methadone (0.2 mg/kg IM or IV) or fentanyl, and move to buprenorphine (0.02 mg/kg) after 24 hours and/or pain scoring.
> - An anticoagulant such as low molecular weight heparin or unfractionated heparin should be started as soon as possible. A factor Xa inhibitor, such as rivaroxaban, may be given when the cat is stable enough to take oral medication.
> - Clopidogrel at a higher loading dose of 75 mg per os and then 18.75 mg PO every 24 hours, when the cat is stable enough to tolerate per os medication.

- For cats in stage B2 (heart disease but no signs of heart failure), administration of pharmaceuticals such as gabapentin or synthetic feline pheromones may be beneficial to help transportation to the practice.
- *In acute cases of CHF* – Check bedding frequently. Minimise stress by having clean bedding ready, and have someone help gently restrain the patient as it is changed.
- Water must be available at all times.
- Regular blood tests should monitor renal and electrolyte parameters to avoid over diuresis.
- Blood pressure should also be monitored regularly to avoid compromising cardiac output.

DRUGS USED IN THE TREATMENT OF ARRHYTHMIAS

There are three types of myocyte in the heart: nodal cells, His-Purkinje cells, and working myocardial cells (Table 7.5).

The rate of atrial and ventricular contraction depends on the electrical properties of the cardiac myocytes, and on the electrical information passed from one region of the heart to another. Antiarrhythmic drugs act not only by suppressing an arrhythmia, but also by aiming to reduce the likelihood of an arrhythmia taking place. This is done by changing the shape of action potentials within cardiac tissue. Cardiac action potential is the activation of myocytes in a precise sequence, in response to a conducted electrical signal, that cause the heart to contract and relax, pumping blood around the body, and refilling. Each of the cells has a different action potential, because of their different function.

Each action potential has five stages (Figure 7.3), and the timing depends upon the permeability of the plasma membrane to potassium, sodium, and calcium ions. It is easiest to look at the phases in three broader groups:

- Phase 0 – Depolarisation
- Phase 1–3 – Repolarisation
- Phase 4 – Resting phase

Table 7.4 Summary of medications used in the treatment of feline heart disease, ATE, and heart failure

Drug	Comment	Form	Dose	Stage recommended for use	Adverse effects
Furosemide	Can be used as with dogs when signs of heart failure are present. The maintenance dose should be titrated based on sleeping respiration rate. The goal of therapy is less than 30 breaths per minute at home when sleeping.	Injectable, liquid, tablet	Loading dose 1–2 mg/kg 0.5–2 mg/kg PO q8–12	C and D	Polyuria, polydipsia, hypokalaemia.
Clopidogrel	Significant left atrial enlargement is present, or after a thrombotic event.	Tablet	18.75 mg/cat PO q24 h,	B, C, and D	Some cats can salivate with administration of clopidogrel. Putting the tablet in a plain gelatine capsule can minimise this.
Pimobendan	Not licenced for use, but may be used by cardiologists.	Tablet	0.625–1.25 mg per cat q12 h	C and D	It is not recommended for cats with outflow tract obstruction.
ACE inhibitors	Sometimes used, but not first line treatment.	Tablet	0.5 mg/kg PO q24 h	C and D	Azotaemia and hypotension. It should not be given if the cat is anorexic.
Torsemide	Can be introduced at stage D, when a cat has become refractory to furosemide. It is only administered once a day, but the longer duration of action may increase renal and electrolyte depletion.	Tablet	0.1–0.2 mg/kg PO q24 h	D	Polyuria, polydipsia, hypokalaemia.
Spironolactone	Used by some cardiologists as a second line diuretic, especially when hypokalaemia is present.	Tablet	1–2 mg/kg PO q12 h to q24 h	D	Reports of ulcerative dermatitis in Maine Coon cats.

Table 7.5 Types of myocyte

Cell type	Function	Location
Nodal cells	Primary pacemakers	In the sinoatrial and atrioventricular nodes
His-Purkinje cells	Rapidly conducting tissue	Throughout the His bundle, the Bundle branches and Purkinje fibre network
Working myocardial cells	Mechanical work	In the atrial and ventricular myocardium

These different phases of the action potential are important because antiarrhythmic drugs are designed to target different stages.

Any drug used in the treatment and management of arrhythmias can have a proarrhythmic effect (worsen the existing arrhythmia), and therefore should be used with caution and close monitoring.

Anti-arrhythmic drugs are split into two groups:

1. Those that treat tachyarrhythmias
2. Those that treat bradyarrhythmias

TACHYARRHYTHMIAS

The primary aim of antiarrhythmic treatment of tachyarrhythmias is to slow the heart rate. This is done by either slowing the depolarisation rate, so targeting phase 0 or 4 of the action potential, or by prolonging repolarisation, targeting phases 1–3. Tachyarrhythmic drugs have been categorised into four different classes, called the Vaughan-Williams

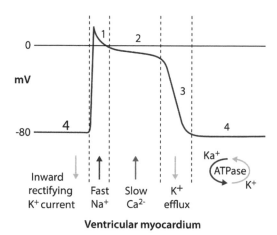

Ventricular myocardium

Figure 7.3 Action potential of a working myocardial cell.

Table 7.6 Vaughan-Williams classification of anti-arrhythmic drugs[5]

Class	Examples	Action	Note
Ia	Procainamide Quinidine	Sodium channel blocker Slows down phase 0 depolarisation and prolongs repolarisation (1–3)	Useful for refractory ventricular arrhythmias and some supraventricular arrhythmias
Ib	Lidocaine Mexilitine	Sodium channel blocker Slows down phase 0 depolarisation in abnormal tissue and prolongs repolarisation (1–3)	Ventricular arrhythmias Occasionally useful in some supraventricular arrhythmias
Ic	Flecainide Encainide	Sodium channel blocker Significant slowing of phase 0 depolarisation	Not used in veterinary medicine
II	Atenolol Propanolol	Anti-adrenergic (beta blockers) drugs – Block transmission of sympathetic nerve fibres	Refractory ventricular arrhythmias Rate control of supraventricular arrhythmias
III	Sotalol Amiodorone	Prolong repolarisation of the atria and ventricles to increase filling time	Used in ventricular and supraventricular arrhythmias
IV	Diltiazem Verapamil	Calcium channel blockers. By inhibiting calcium in the pacemaker cells, depolarisation is slowed	Rate control of supraventricular arrhythmias

classification (Table 7.6). Class one blocks sodium channels and has been subdivided in to three separate groups.

LIDOCAINE

Lidocaine (class Ib) is the most commonly used drug in the treatment of tachyarrhythmias because it works quickly and has a wide range of use. It should be used intravenously (IV). It has a short half-life of approximately an hour, so boluses may be needed, or a continuous rate infusion (CRI).

DOSE

Dogs – 2 mg/kg bolus, up to 6–8 mg/kg over ten minutes. It should be administered IV, over 1–2 minutes. Each bolus should be given a couple of minutes to act. CRIs are indicated at a lower dose of 25–100 micrograms/kg/minute.
Cats – Should be used with caution as cats are more prone to neurotoxic effects. 0.5 mg/kg bolus, up to 2 mg/kg bolus.
Adverse effects – Neurotoxicity, such as seizures and tremors, and gastrotoxicity, i.e., vomiting and diarrhoea. Adverse cardiac effects are rare.

MEXILITINE

Mexilitine is also a class Ib antiarrhythmic drug. It is used for chronic management of ventricular arrhythmias.

DOSE

Dogs – 4–8 mg/kg every 8–12 hours per os. It must be administered with food or on a
    full stomach due to the common gastrotoxic effects.
Cats – Not recommended for use in cats.
Adverse effects – Nausea and vomiting.

BETA ADRENERGIC BLOCKERS

Beta adrenergic, or beta blockers as they are more commonly known, are class II drugs. They are used to treat atrial tachyarrhythmias by slowing conduction through the atrioventricular (AV) node, which in turn, slows the ventricular rate. It is used in patients with atrial fibrillation. Atenolol is the most commonly used beta adrenergic blocker and is also used to treat hypertension.

DOSE

Atenolol – 0.2–1.5 mg/kg in dogs and 0.5–3 mg/kg in cats.
Adverse effects – Beta blockers can reduce contractility and ventricular relaxation, and
    therefore not indicated for use in patients that have systolic dysfunction or poorly
    controlled CHF. It can also cause hypotension.

SOTALOL

Sotalol is a class III antiarrhythmic with some class II beta blocking properties. It is primarily used to treat ventricular arrhythmias, but is sometimes used in cases of atrial fibrillation. There are different dose rates, depending upon which arrhythmias are being treated. It is sometimes used in cats.

Adverse effects: Because of the beta blocking effects, it should not be used in cases with systolic dysfunction or poorly controlled CHF. It can cause bradyarrhythmias and have proarrhythmic effects.

DILTIAZEM

Diltiazem is a class IV antiarrhythmic. It is a calcium channel blocker that targets the sinus rate and AV node conduction. It is used to treat atrial tachycardias, and can come in different forms. Sustained release versions mean less frequent dosing, which may be preferential in cats. It is available in injectable and tablet form.

ADVERSE EFFECTS

Accurate dosing is important because it is generally well tolerated. At increased doses, it can exasperate CHF by cause hypotension and decrease cardiac output. It can also cause bradyarrhythmias.

DIGOXIN

Digoxin is not included in the Vaughan-Williams classification, but is a commonly used drug to treat atrial fibrillation. It is a digitalis glycoside and is the oldest antiarrhythmic drug, originating from the Digitalis plant. Its main actions are to inhibit sodium pump action, activate parasympathetic tone and inhibit sympathetic tone, which slow ventricular rate.

Dosing accuracy is very important with digoxin, and should be calculated on lean bodyweight. It has a very narrow therapeutic window, meaning toxicity can easily occur. Toxicity is more likely to occur with renal insufficiency or hypokalaemia, so electrolyte and renal monitoring is vital, especially if the patient is also being treated with diuretics. Peak serum concentrations occur between 5 and 7 days, and accurate dosing is monitored on clinical signs and via trough serum digoxin levels (more than 8 hours post pill), aiming at a concentration of 0.6–1.1 ng/ml. This means that serum digoxin levels should also be monitored regularly. It is mainly prescribed twice daily in dogs, but can be used in cats, every 48 hours.

ADVERSE EFFECTS

Central nervous system effects – Depressed mentation, anorexia, vomiting, and
   diarrhoea.
Cardiac effects – Tachy or bradyarrhythmias.

BRADYARRHYTHMIAS

In small animal medicine, bradyarrhythmias are most commonly encountered as a result of general anaesthesia, sedation, or high vagal tone. Treatment is rarely indicated further than reversing the actions of the drug (such as reversing medetomidine) or treating the underlying condition. On the rare occasions where bradyarrhythmias require treatment, it can be because they are:

- Electrically unstable, where sudden death is possible
- Compromising haemodynamic function, causing hypoperfusion, and signs of CHF

TREATMENT

Bradyarrhythmias that require treatment are high grade atrioventricular (AV) block, sinus node dysfunction and atrial standstill. If there is an underlying cause, this needs to be treated first. For example, hyperkalaemia (seen accompanying Addisonian crisis or oliguria) should be rectified. For cases of high grade AV block or sinus node dysfunction, pacemaker implantation may be the most effective treatment. Pacemakers can be placed in dogs and cats.

If drugs are used in the treatment of bradyarrhythmias, the aim is to increase heart rate and conduction from the atria to the ventricles, by stimulating the sinoatrial (SA) and AV nodes. They are indicated for use in arrhythmias such as AV block and sinus arrest. Table 7.7 summarizes the drugs used to treat bradyarrhytmias.

Table 7.7 Drugs used in the management of bradyarrhythmias

Class	Example	Action
Anticholinergic	Atropine	Inhibit effects of vagal tone
	Glycopyrrolate	
	Propantheline bromide	
Sympathomimetic	Beta-adrenergic agonists	Mimic the effects of sympathetic tone
	• Terbutaline	
	• Isoproterenol	
	Methylxanthines	
	• Theophylline	
	• Etamiphylline	
	• Aminophylline	

KEY POINTS

- Any drug can have an adverse effect, therefore cardiac patients need close monitoring.
- Cardiac medications need to be assessed regularly, either by blood sampling, blood pressure measurement and/or 24 hour ECG.
- Cats may require CHF treatment, and antithrombotics to prevent or treat thrombus formation.
- When adding more medications, the welfare of the patient needs to be taken into consideration, and the cost to the owner.

FURTHER READING

Ferasin L, DeFrancesco T (2015). Management of acute heart failure in cats. *Journal of Veterinary Cardiology.* 17: S173–S189.

Gordon S; Côté, E (2015). Pharmacology of feline cardiomyopathy: chronic management of heart failure. *Journal of Veterinary Cardiology.* 17: S159–172.

REFERENCES

1. Summerfield NJ, Boswood A, O'Grady MR, Gordon SG, Dukes-McEwan J, Oyama MA, Smith S, Patterson M, French AT, Culshaw GJ, Braz-Ruivo L, Estrada A, O'Sullivan ML, Loureiro J, Willis R, Watson P (2012). Efficacy of pimobendan in the prevention of congestive heart failure or sudden death in Doberman Pinschers with preclinical dilated cardiomyopathy (The PROTECT study). *Journal of Veterinary Internal Medicine.* 26: 1337–1349.
2. Boswood A, Häggström J, Gordon SG, Wess G, Stepien R, Oyama MA, Keene BW, Bonagura J, MacDonald KS, Patterson M, Smith S, Fox PR, Sanderson K, Woolley R, Szartmári V, Menaut P, Church WM, O'Sullivan ML, Jaudon J-P, Kresken J-G, Rush J, Barrett KA, Rosenthal SL, Saunders AB, Ljunvall I, Deinert M, Bomassi E, Estrada AH, Fernandez

Del Palacio MJ, Moise NS, Abbott JA, Fujii Y, Spier A, Luethy MW, Santilli RA, Uechi M, Tidholm A, Watson P (2016). Effect of pimobendan in dogs with preclinical myxomatous valve disease and cardiomegaly: The EPIC study – A randomized clinical trial. *Journal of Veterinary Internal Medicine.* 30(6): 1765–1779.

3. Hogan DF, Fox PR, Jacob K, Keene B, Laste NJ, Rosenthal S, Sederquist K, Weng HY (2015). Secondary prevention of cardiogenic arterial thromboembolism in the cat: The double-blind, randomized, positive-controlled feline arterial thromboembolism; clopidogrel vs. aspirin trial (FAT CAT). *Journal of Veterinary Cardiology.* 17: S306–317.

4. Luis Fuentes V, Abbott J, Chetboul V, Côté E, Fox PR, Häggström J, Kittleson MD, Schober K, Stern JA (2020). ACVIM consensus statement guidelines for the classification, diagnosis, and management of cardiomyopathies in cats. *Journal of Veterinary Internal Medicine.* 34(3): 1062–1077.

5. Dennis S (2010). Antiarrhythmic therapies. In *BSAVA Manual of Canine and Feline Cardiorespiratory Medicine*, 2nd edition. British Small Animal Veterinary Association, Gloucester.

8

Cardiac emergencies – First aid

This chapter focuses on emergency presentation of patients suffering from heart failure, complications arising from heart disease or life threatening arrhythmias. The pathophysiology of these presentations is discussed in other chapters. The emergency situations that are covered are:

1. *Respiratory distress* – Congestive heart failure (CHF), where fluid has accumulated and restricts normal oxygenation.
2. *Collapse* – Forward or output failure, where the heart cannot pump sufficient blood to meet the body's demands.
3. *Feline aortic thromboembolism (ATE)* – A clot that has caused partial paresis or paralysis. As well as acute pain, heart failure may also be present.
4. Life threatening arrhythmias.

It is important to remember that these events can be very traumatising for the owner. For some, it may be the inevitable they knew was coming, but with others, particularly cat owners and certain arrhythmias, an emergency is the first indication that their pet has heart disease.

This chapter details the approach veterinary nurses should take when a patient attends their practice, or emergency room. The most important thing is to reduce stress to the patient to an absolute minimum. This might conflict with trying to get a diagnosis, but it is the nurse's role to be the advocate for their patient. Often when nursing patients with heart failure and/or ATE, less is more. The aims of emergency treatment are to

- Promote ventricular filling
- Alleviate CHF signs
- Prevent thromboembolism
- Control arrhythmias if present

FROM INITIAL CLIENT CONTACT (TELEPHONE)

- Prepare an oxygen supply. Ideally, this should be in a quiet place, but one that allows easy observation. The method of oxygen supplementation should not stress the patient. If the patient will not tolerate flow by, then do not pursue it.
- Ensure that furosemide is ready, and that it is in date.
- Prepare the kennel or place where oxygen will be provided. A vetbed is ideal as it will remove urine away from the patient.
- Depending upon the nature of the emergency, prepare equipment for intravenous catheterisation.

ON ARRIVAL AT THE CLINIC

- A veterinary surgeon should be contacted immediately.
- The patient should be carried or placed on a trolley to transport from the door/car to the oxygen supply.
- Ask the owner to remain in reception whilst emergency work can be initiated. If there is staff available to be with owners, take as many details as possible, for example a relevant history, including what was happening when the event took place, and current medication.
- Depending upon the stability of the patient, an accurate weight is desirable but not essential. A guess from an experienced team member will suffice until the patient is stable.
- Whilst oxygen is being provided, the veterinary surgeon should auscultate and examine the patient, feeling for pulses at the same time. Box 8.1 outlines what may be heard on auscultation and where.
- Table 8.1 summarises treatment by presentation. However, all cases should receive oxygen supplementation, in as stress-free manner as possible.
- Minimal stress. Sedation may be necessary in some cases where patients are very distressed. Butorphanol intramuscularly (IM) is most commonly recommended at a dose rate of 0.2–0.4 mg/kg.

AFTER INITIAL STABILISATION

- Access to plentiful water and checked regularly for urination.
- If changing bedding, stress should be minimised. Be organised, and if available, use an assistant to remove the bed and place a clean one.
- Intravenous access (IV) can now be gained (if not already), as long as it is not stressful to the patient. If it is upsetting the patient, do it in stages. For example, clip leg, rest, clean, place catheter and secure, rest, bandage and rest. Local anaesthetic cream can be used, but be mindful of how many times the patient is being handled. Less is more with cardiac patients.
- Blood samples may be required, as a minimum for renal and electrolytes parameters. This would be to assess the effect of diuresis. Over diuresis can cause hypokalaemia.
- Blood pressure may also be required to assess cardiac output. This should be done as calmly as possible.
- Allow the patient time to rest between tests.

BOX 8.1: Auscultation and physical findings in a cardiac emergency

- *Pulmonary crackles* – Indicate pulmonary oedema. These are heard louder over dorsal lung fields.
- *Dull heart sounds* – Indicates an effusion in the thoracic cavity, either pleural or pericardial. This is heard more ventrally.
- Alternatively, if the patient is collapsed, an arrhythmia may be present. If this is the case, the patient may have poor or absent pulses, cold extremities, or pallor.
- If a cat has had a thrombotic event, it may be vocalising and be extremely painful, showing obvious signs of paralysis.

Table 8.1 Presentation and emergency treatment

Pulmonary oedema	Pleural effusion	Collapse	ATE
Furosemide either intravenously (IV), if access can be gained without stress, or intramuscularly (IM) until IV access can be achieved This can be given as boluses at 2 mg/kg up to 8 mg/kg in 4 hours, or as a continuous rate infusion (CRI). Monitor respiratory rate (RR) and respiratory effort (RE)	Furosemide either IV or IM Prepare thoracocentesis equipment (see kit list)	IV catheter placed. If caused by an arrhythmia, attach ECG and treat accordingly. Ventricular tachycardia can be treated with lidocaine at a 2 mg/kg bolus IV, it should be administered intravenously, over 1–2 minutes up to 6–8 mg/kg over ten minutes. Each bolus should be given a couple of minutes to act. If due to acute decompensated heart failure: Blood pressure measurements Administration of pimobendan (0.25–0.3 mg/kg q12) and furosemide as required.	Analgesia. Either methadone (0.02 mg/kg IM/IV) or fentanyl are recommended. Furosemide if CHF present also Anticoagulant therapy to be initiated as early as possible. If CHF present, oxygen therapy and diuresis (either IM or IV) should be administered. Check bedding, keep warm and comfortable. Monitor vital signs, demeanour Caution with warming patient if hypothermic to avoid vasodilation. Do not use direct heat sources to avoid scalds. Room temperature is sufficient.

It can be difficult to distinguish between respiratory disease and congestive heart failure in emergency situations, but until the veterinary surgeon has made a diagnosis, emergency care is similar, supplemental oxygen and minimal handling. A one off dose of furosemide will not harm a patient suffering from respiratory disease.

ACUTE MANAGEMENT OF RESPIRATORY DISTRESS

If the patient presents with pulmonary oedema, furosemide should be given, and if not responding, a continuous rate infusion can be attached. Centesis is not possible because the fluid has accumulated in the lungs. For pleural or pericardial effusion, see guides below.

THORACOCENTESIS

Thoracocentesis is a surgical procedure that involves the removal of fluid from the thorax using a needle. It is more commonly performed in cats diagnosed with CHF, and can significantly improve oxygenation thereby easing respiratory effort, and decrease the respiratory rate. Opiate sedation may be necessary. Butorphanol is often used in these cases. Figure 8.1 lists equipment that could be kept in a box ready for when it is needed.

HOW TO PREPARE A PATIENT FOR THORACOCENTESIS

Patient should be in sternal recumbency. Gentle restraint may be all that is necessary (Figure 8.2).

Clip the thorax – The catheter will be inserted between the 7th to 9th intercostal spaces. Clip the ventral two-thirds of the chest. The veterinary surgeon may specify which side they want prepared, or they may require both sides to be clipped. Often pleural fluid will form in pockets, so both sides will be tapped.

Prepare the thorax using a chlorhexidine solution and surgical spirit (Figure 8.3). This may need to be done around the veterinary surgeon visualising the area using ultrasound guidance.

Comfy bed for the patient to sit on
Clippers
Prep solution and swabs
Surgical spirit
Sterile gloves for the veterinary surgeon
Ultrasound machine ready, if available, and ultrasound gel
Appropriate sized butterfly catheters (cats) or intravenous catheters (dogs)
Three way tap
10 or 20 ml syringe for cats, 20–60 ml for dogs
Collecting dish or jug
Ethylenediaminetetraacetic acid (EDTA) tube for cell counts
Plain tube for culture and cytology

Local anaesthesia may be required, but many veterinary surgeons find it unnecessary.

Figure 8.1 Equipment needed for thoracocentesis. A box could be used with equipment prepared, and a checklist.

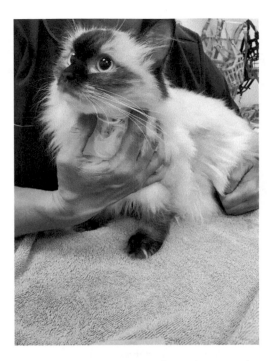

Figure 8.2 Photograph showing gentle restraint of a cat about to undergo thoracocentesis.

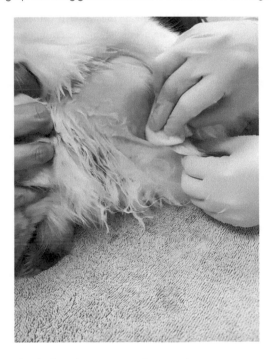

Figure 8.3 Preparation before thoracocentesis procedure.

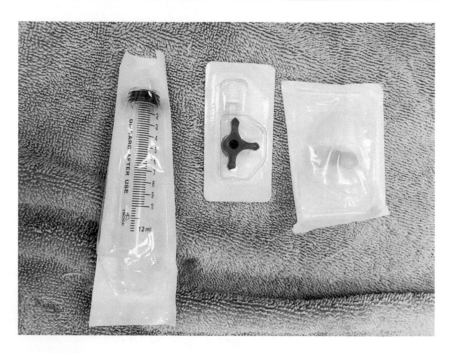

Figure 8.4 Syringe, butterfly catheter and three way tap.

The veterinary surgeon aseptically connects the butterfly catheter to the three way tap and syringe (Figure 8.4) and inserts the needle along the cranial edge of the rib. Gentle pressure is placed on the syringe and fluid removed (Figure 8.5), or in the absence of fluid, the needle is repositioned.

Samples may be needed for analysis, so ensure EDTA and plain tubes are filled aseptically.

The role of the nurse is to restrain the patient, minimise stress, and assist with the procedure. When the veterinary surgeon has finished, let the patient rest. Often when thoracocentesis is performed, the nurse restraining can feel the cat 'sigh' as the lungs can expand fully.

Whilst respiration will have improved, it is important to continue minimising stress and keep patient handling to a minimum. Administer medication as directed, encourage the patient to eat, and provide easy access to litter tray and water.

PERICARDIOCENTESIS

Pericardiocentesis may be necessary for patients with large amounts of pericardial fluid that is compromising cardiac function. Due to the risk of complications, sedation is often required. Figure 8.6 lists equipment that might be needed for pericardiocentesis.

HOW TO PREPARE A PATIENT FOR PERICARDIOCENTESIS

The patient should lie in left lateral recumbency, and preferably, attached to an electrocardiograph (ECG). Sedation may be needed.

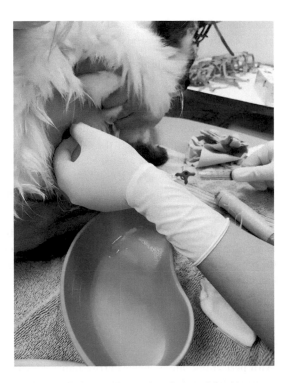

Figure 8.5 Thoracocentesis being performed and pleural fluid being removed.

Comfy bed for patient to sit on
Clippers
Prep solution and swabs
Surgical spirit
Sterile gloves for the veterinary surgeon
Ultrasound machine ready, if available, and ultrasound gel
ECG machine connected to patient
Appropriate sized intravenous catheter or jugular catheter
Three-way tap
Extension set to allow distance from the patient and the operator
Appropriate size syringe
Collecting dish or jug
EDTA tube for cell counts
Plain tube for culture and cytology

Local anaesthesia may be required.

Figure 8.6 Equipment needed for pericardiocentesis.

Clip a large area of the right chest wall. The catheter will be inserted between the 5th and 6th intercostal space at the costrochondral junction.

- Prepare the thorax using a chlorhexidine solution and surgical spirit. This may need to be done around the veterinary surgeon visualising the area using ultrasound guidance.
- The veterinary surgeon will either use an over-the-needle catheter, such as an IV catheter, or a through-the-needle jugular catheter, using the Seldinger technique.
- The veterinary surgeon aseptically connects the catheter to the three way tap and syringe and inserts the needle along the cranial edge of the rib, or places a catheter using the Seldinger technique.
- Samples may be needed for analysis, so ensure EDTA and plain tubes are filled aseptically.

The role of the nurse is to restrain the patient, minimise stress, and assist with the procedure. This includes opening and passing equipment in an aseptic manner and monitoring the ECG during the procedure. When the veterinary surgeon has finished, let the patient rest. Even a small amount of fluid removed can significantly reduce intrapericardial pressure and improve the status of the patient. Depending upon the size of the patient, the amount of fluid removed can vary between 10 ml and two litres.

COMPLICATIONS

Risks associated with pericardiocentesis include arrhythmias which can be life threatening, cardiac puncture, haemorrhage, infection, or tumour laceration. If ventricular arrhythmias occur during the procedure, alert the veterinary surgeon. It will often resolve once the catheter is repositioned.

COLLAPSE

There are a few reasons why a patient may present collapsed. For example:

- A sudden deterioration in advanced heart disease, such as a ruptured chordae tendineae in a dog with myxomatous mitral valve disease
- A dog with dilated cardiomyopathy developing an arrhythmia
- A cat with severe cardiomyopathy
- A dog or cat with a sudden onset arrhythmia, such as ventricular tachycardia

COLLAPSE RESULTING FROM SEVERE DISEASE

In cases where patients have deteriorated acutely, there may not have been time for compensatory mechanisms to activate. This is called decompensated heart failure. Management goals are to maximise haemodynamic function and improve hypoxaemia. Neutralising neurohormonal activity, such as the administration of furosemide, may be counterproductive at this point, as arterial pressures may be relying on this fluid volume, and therefore removing it could be deleterious.

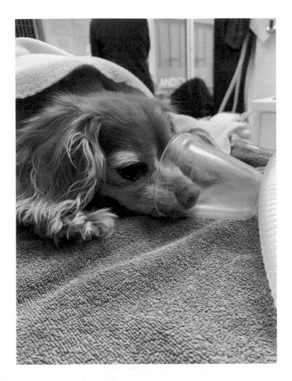

Figure 8.7 Collapsed patient receiving supplemental oxygen via mask.

As with CHF, reducing stress and providing oxygen are crucial (Figure 8.7). Positive inotropes such as pimobendan might be used to improve ventricular contraction, at a dose rate of 0.25–0.3 mg/kg twice daily. Arterial dilators such as dobutamine may be used with extreme caution using constant ECG monitoring and regular measurement of blood pressure.

It goes without saying that treating patients at this stage of cardiac disease have a poor prognosis. Therefore, along with close nursing of the patient, nurses may also be required to support owners making a difficult decision.

COLLAPSE RESULTING FROM ARRHYTHMIA

If the patient has collapsed as the result of an arrhythmia, then the following procedure should be followed:

- Notify a veterinary surgeon immediately
- Attach an ECG
- Place an IV catheter, ensuring patency

Upon veterinary surgeon instruction and diagnosis of the arrhythmia, prepare emergency drugs. If there are underlying causes these should be treated, such as hypokalaemia and hypomagnesaemia. Table 8.2 summarises treatment and drug intervention that may be required for emergency arrhythmias.

Table 8.2 Summary of treatment for arrhythmias

Ventricular tachycardia	Boluses of lidocaine at 2 mg/kg IV given over 1–2 minutes. Repeat as necessary up to 8 mg/kg. In some cases of ventricular tachycardia, sotalol may be used at 1 mg/kg IV given over 3–5 minutes. If patient deteriorates, prepare for cardiopulmonary resuscitation and defibrillation (if available) (Figure 8.8).
Atrial standstill	Measure serum potassium. Hyperkalaemia – Intravenous fluid therapy 0.9% NaCl and IV calcium gluconate.
AV block (high grade 2nd or 3rd degree)	If heart rate less than 40 beats/minute, rule out other possible causes. Pacemaker implantation may be considered
Atrial fibrillation	May be sudden onset if severe disease is already present. CHF should be treated and digoxin used (3–5 micrograms/kg, q12h PO) to slow ventricular rate. If no disease is present, and left atrial size is normal for the breed, electric cardioversion could be considered.

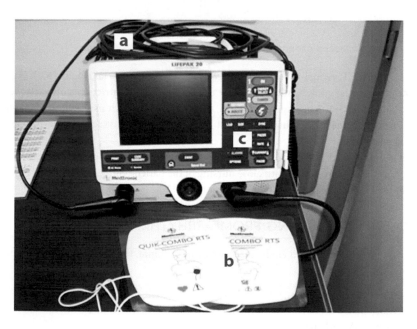

Figure 8.8 Machine capable of defibrillation (paddles on top), temporary pacing using transthoracic adhesive pads, and electrical cardioversion to convert atrial fibrillation to sinus rhythm. (a) Paddles for defibrillation; (b) Transthoracic pacing pads; (c) control panel.

If the patient returns to sinus rhythm, or the rate is restored to normal for that species and breed, caution must still be exercised with the patient afterwards. If the underlying cause was not found, it is possible that with stress or exertion, the arrhythmia may return. Also, the patient is likely to be fatigued, and will need rest.

Refer to Chapter 5 for RECOVER CPR guidelines.

KEY POINTS

- Reduce stress and minimise handling.
- Monitor from a distance where possible, taking regular respiratory rates, or leaving an ECG connected.
- Any form of exercise (even toileting) is only to be considered once the patient has stabilised.
- Less is more in cases that are life threatening. IM furosemide is adequate.
- Any cat presenting with an ATE needs adequate pain relief.

FURTHER READING

Ferasin L, DeFrancesco T, 2015. Management of acute heart failure in cats. *Journal of Veterinary Cardiology.* 17: S173–S189.

Keene BW, Atkins CE, Bonagura JD, Fox PR, Häggström J, Luis Fuentes V, Oyama MA, Rush JE, Stepien R, Uechi M, 2019. ACVIM consensus guidelines for the diagnosis and treatment of myxomatous mitral valve disease in dogs. *Journal of Veterinary Internal Medicine.* 33(3):1127–1140.

Luis Fuentes V, Abbott J, Chetboul V, Côté E, Fox PR, Häggström J, Kittleson MD, Schober K, Stern JA (2020). ACVIM consensus statement guidelines for the classification, diagnosis, and management of cardiomyopathies in cats. *Journal of Veterinary Internal Medicine.* 34(3): 1062–1077.

Glossary

Abdominocentesis   Removing fluid from the abdomen using a needle or catheter aseptically. Can be performed for therapeutic or diagnostic reasons.

Action potential   In cardiology terms, an action potential is a change in voltage across the cell membrane of a myocyte. It is caused by the movement of charged atoms and creates the electrical impulse that initiates muscle contraction.

Acute   Sudden onset.

Addisonian crisis   Life threatening condition where hyperkalaemia can cause a significant decrease in heart rate.

Adrenergic system   *See sympathetic nervous system.*

Anticoagulant drugs   A group of drugs that slow down the clotting process, by reducing fibrin formation. Examples are heparin and warfarin.

Antiplatelet drugs   A group of drugs that prevent platelets from clumping together to form a clot. Examples are aspirin and clopidogrel.

Anxiolytic   Drug used to reduce anxiety.

Aorta   One of the two great arteries, that transports oxygenated blood from the left ventricle around the head and body

Aortic stenosis   Narrowing of the aorta, either at the level of the aortic valves, above (supravalvular), or below (subvalvular).

Aortic thromboembolism (ATE)   A blood clot within the aorta, that is often found at the bifurcation of the aorta, at the femoral arteries. A condition that particularly affects cats. Also known as feline aortic thromboembolism and saddle thrombus.

Aortic valve   One of the semilunar valves. The aortic valve is located between the left ventricle and aorta, and closes after systole, to prevent the backflow of blood.

Arrhythmia   Abnormal heart rhythm. An arrhythmia can be fast, slow or irregular.

Artefact   Interference found on an ECG trace. Can be caused by electrical equipment, panting, respiration or purring.

Ascites   Abnormal fluid accumulation in the abdomen.

Atrioventricular (AV) node   Key part of the conduction system of the heart that lies to the right of the atrioventricular junction. It acts as a relay for the electrical impulse, coordinating contraction of the atria and ventricles. It consists of specialised cells.

Atrioventricular valves   Collective term used for describing the mitral and tricuspid valves. The atrioventricular valves are located between the atria and the ventricles.

Atrium (pleural atria)   Upper chambers of the heart. The atria receive blood from the vena cava and pulmonary veins. Blood crosses the atrioventricular valves and into the ventricles. They are smaller than the bottom chambers as they do not perform the same workload.

Auscultation   Term used to describe listening to the heart and lungs with a stethoscope.

Azotaemia   Increased blood urea nitrogen and creatinine.

Balloon valvuloplasty   Procedure that is used to widen a narrowed heart valve.

Bradyarrhythmia   Arrhythmia that is slower than normal.

Bradycardia   Slower than normal heart rate.

Cardiac cachexia   Loss of muscle or lean body mass associated with heart failure.

Cardiac disease   *See heart disease.*

Cardiomyopathy   Disease of the heart muscle. Most commonly it is an acquired heart disease. Examples are hypertrophic cardiomyopathy or dilated cardiomyopathy.

Cardiac output   Volume of blood pumped from the heart per minute.

Cardiac tamponade   Abnormal accumulation of fluid in the pericardium that increases pressure on the heart chambers, and restricts cardiac function.

Carotid arteries   Two arteries that provide oxygenated blood to the brain, head, and neck.

Centesis   Removing fluid from a cavity, using a needle aseptically. Can be performed for therapeutic or diagnostic reasons.

Chordae tendineae   Strands of connective tissue that connect the heart valves to papillary muscles in the ventricle.

Chronic   Long term.

Chronic mitral valve fibrosis   *See myxomatous mitral valve disease.*

Chronic degenerative valvular disease   Degenerative disease of both the mitral and tricuspid valves.

Chronic valvular disease   *See chronic degenerative valvular disease.*

Compensatory mechanisms   Compensatory mechanisms are activated when blood pressure falls. In acute cases, this can be lifesaving. In cardiac terms, these mechanisms are chronically activated causing damaging side effects. The compensatory mechanisms are the sympathetic nervous system and the renin angiotensin and aldosterone system.

Concentric   A circular form within another circular shape, such as a circular lesion within the aorta.

Congestive heart failure (CHF)   When clinical signs of increased tissue water and/or decreased tissue perfusion are present. Occurs as a result of heart disease. The more common presentation of heart failure.

Coronary arteries   Two arteries that supply the heart with oxygenated blood.

Contractility   Pumping ability of cardiac muscle.

Degenerative mitral valve disease   *See myxomatous mitral valve disease.*

Depolarisation   In conduction terms, as the electrical current passes through the cardiac muscle and makes the myocardium contract. This is when blood is forcibly ejected in systole.

Diastole   Phase of the cardiac cycle when the heart muscle relaxes. It allows the heart chambers to fill with blood.

Dilated cardiomyopathy (DCM)   Acquired heart disease that is defined by cardiac enlargement because of weakened ventricular myocardial function. The ventricles stretch and become dilated over time. In severe cases, can lead to heart failure, and/or arrhythmias.

Diuresis   Group of drugs used to remove excess fluid via an increase in urine output.

Echocardiography   Ultrasound of the heart, allowing observation of individual heart chambers, valves, blood flow patterns and functionality.

Electrocardiograph (ECG)   Method used to record the conduction system of the heart. Shows heart rate and rhythm.

Endocardiosis   *See chronic degenerative valvular disease.*

Feline aortic thromboembolism (FATE)   *See aortic thromboembolism.*

Fibrillation   Rapid and irregular small movements of fibres causing a lack of coordination in electrical conduction.
   Atrial fibrillation is commonly seen with moderate to severe heart disease. Ventricular fibrillation is life threatening.

Forward failure   Insufficient cardiac output to maintain blood pressure. Also known as output failure.

Gallop rhythm   An additional heart sound to the normal 'lub dub'. Called a gallop rhythm because it can sound like a horse running. It is caused by stiff ventricles.

Heart disease   Abnormality of cardiac structure or function.

Heart murmur   Any abnormal heart sound of prolonged duration. It can occur because of an abnormal valve, the narrowing of a major artery, or because the heart is having to handle more blood quicker than normal.

Heart failure   Can refer to congestive heart failure or forward heart failure.

Holter monitor   Ambulatory ECG that can be attached to a patient to record heart rate and rhythm continuously. Often used for 24 hours but can be used for longer.

Hyperkalaemia   Increased potassium in the blood. Can cause bradycardia.

Hypertension   Increased blood pressure.

Hypertrophy   Increased muscle size.

Hypertrophic cardiomyopathy   Acquired heart disease that is defined by an in increase in cardiac muscle. The ventricles become thick and stiff over time. In severe cases, can lead to heart failure, and/or arrhythmias. Most commonly seen in cats.

Hypoxaemia   Insufficient oxygen in the blood. Can be seen in some cases of heart failure.

Hypoxia   Insufficient oxygen in the tissue. Can be seen in some cases of heart failure.

Ischaemia   Sudden lack of blood supply to an organ or tissue. Often seen as a consequence of a thrombotic event.

Limb contracture   Inability to move limb properly, because of tightness or stiffness. Seen in cats after a thrombotic event.

Mitral regurgitation   Blood flow that leaks through the mitral valve, back into the left atrium, because the valve leaflets do not close properly.

Mitral valve   One of the atrioventricular valves. The mitral valve is located between the left atrium and left ventricle. Closes at the end of diastole, and the beginning of systole.

Mitral valve disease   *See myxomatous mitral valve disease.*

Myxomatous mitral valve disease   Chronic disease that affects the left atrioventricular valve. Degenerative changes may occur quickly or slowly. Some cases will develop left sided congestive heart failure, some severe cases may also develop right sided congestive heart failure as well. Most commonly seen in dogs.

   Also called chronic mitral valve fibrosis, degenerative mitral valve disease, mitral valve disease.

Output failure   *See forward failure.*

Pallor   Pale appearance.

Paresis   Either partial paralysis or difficult to move voluntarily.

Paradoxical breathing   Exaggerated breathing pattern that involves the thorax and abdomen moving at opposite times. Often seen with respiratory disease or fluid accumulation in the pleural or abdominal cavity.

Paralysis   Partial or total loss of function or sensation in the affected area.

Parasympathetic nervous system   Opposite of the sympathetic nervous system. The parasympathetic nervous system allows for relaxation and conservation of energy.

Patent ductus arteriosus   Persistent connection between the aorta and pulmonary artery. Ordinarily, this should close at the time of birth, or shortly after.

Pericardial effusion   Abnormal fluid accumulation in the pericardial sac. Can cause cardiac tamponade.

Pericardiocentesis   Removing fluid from the pericardial sac, using a needle or catheter aseptically.

Phenotype   In genetics, a set of observable and measurable traits.

Pleural effusion   Abnormal fluid accumulation in the thoracic cavity. Can be cardiac in origin, but can have other causes, such as neoplasia.

Precordial thrill   Vibration that can be felt through skin and fur.

Positive inotropes   Group of drugs that help contractility of the ventricles.

Proarrhythmic   Drug therapy that worsens existing arrhythmia.

Pulmonary artery   One of the two great arteries, that pushes deoxygenated blood from the right ventricle to the lungs for oxygenation.

Pulmonary hypertension   Increased pressure in the pulmonary artery. Occurs either because of respiratory disease, or as a response to high left sided cardiac pressures.

Pulmonary oedema   Abnormal fluid accumulation in the lungs. Often caused by heart failure, but can have other causes such as pneumonia.

Pulmonic stenosis   Narrowing of the pulmonary artery, either at the level of the aortic valves, or above (supravalvular) or below (subvalvular).

Pulmonic valve   One of the semilunar valves. The pulmonic valve is located between the right ventricle and pulmonary artery, and closes after systole, to prevent the backflow of blood.

Pulse deficit   Identified when there is a heart contraction heard on auscultation, but no corresponding pulse is felt. Occurs often because of an ineffective contraction. Can indicate an arrhythmia.

Natriuresis   Removal of sodium through urine.

Neurohormonal mechanisms   Compensatory mechanism. Also known as the renin angiotensin aldosterone system.

Refractory   Stage of heart failure that no longer responds to standard treatment.

Renin angiotensin aldosterone system   Compensatory mechanism. Also known as the neurohormonal system. Its main actions are to constrict blood vessels and retain sodium and water, in an attempt to improve and increase cardiac output.

Reperfusion injury Can occur after a thrombotic event, when tissue perfusion and oxygen supply are restored to an area of ischaemia. The effects of reperfusion can be more disastrous than the initial ischaemia. Clinical signs include hyperkalaemia, arrhythmia, depression and sudden death.

Repolarisation In conduction terms, occurs when the myocardium relaxes, and repositions ready to contract again. Occurs during diastole.

Respiratory sinus arrhythmia A relatively common finding in dogs, especially fit and healthy ones. The heart rate increases during inspiration and pauses during expiration. Also seen when patients are under general anaesthesia.

Saddle thrombus *See aortic thromboembolism.*

Semilunar Collective term used for describing the aortic and pulmonic valves. The aortic valve is between the left ventricle and aorta, the pulmonic valve between the right ventricle and pulmonary artery.

Sinoatrial (SA) node Key part of the conduction system of the heart that acts as the pacemaker of the heart. It is situated in the right atrium.

Sinus Normal.

Sinus arrhythmia *See respiratory sinus arrhythmia.*

Spontaneous echo contrast (SEC) Seen in cardiac chambers on echocardiography and indicates blood stasis. Is a known precursor to thrombus formation.

Smoke Name often used to describe the appearance of spontaneous echo contrast.

Stenosis Narrowing.

Systole Phase of the cardiac cycle when the heart muscle contracts, ejecting blood from the ventricles.

Systolic anterior motion Occurs when the anterior mitral valve leaflet is pulled back into the left ventricular outflow tract (the point where the left ventricle ends, and the aorta starts) during systole. The valve causes an obstruction to blood flow, causing a heart murmur. The murmur often increases in intensity with increases in heart rate.

Syncope Fainting.

Sympathetic nervous system Compensatory mechanism. Also known as the adrenergic system. It is responsible for the fight or flight response, increasing adrenaline and noradrenaline. Its main actions are to increase heart rate and the force of ventricular contraction, and constrict blood vessels, in an attempt to improve and increase cardiac output.

Tachycardia Faster than normal heart rate.

Tamponade *See cardiac tamponade.*

Tricuspid valve One of the atrioventricular valves. The tricuspid valve is located between the right atrium and right ventricle.

Thoracocentesis Removing fluid from the thorax using a needle or catheter aseptically. Can be performed for therapeutic or diagnostic reasons.

Thromboembolism *See aortic thromboembolism.*

Thrombus Blood clot.

Valvuloplasty *See balloon valvuloplasty.*

Vasoconstriction Narrowing of blood vessel muscle walls.

Vasodilation Widening of blood vessel muscle walls.

Venepuncture Taking a blood sample.

Vena cava Two large veins, the superior and inferior vena cava, that carry deoxygenated blood to the right atrium.

Index

Note: Page references in *italics* refer to figures and in **bold** refer to tables.

A

Acquired heart disease in cats, 33–47
    aetiology, 34–38
    clinical signs of, 38–47
    findings on auscultation, 39–41
    nursing and treatment of, 41–47
    prognosis of, 47
    signalment, 33–34
    terminology, 33–38
Acquired heart disease in dogs, 15–30
    dilated cardiomyopathy
        (DCM), 25–29
    myxomatous mitral valve disease
        (MMVD), 15–25
    pericardial disease, 30
Acute management of respiratory
        distress, 122–126
    pericardiocentesis, 124–126
    thoracocentesis, 122–124, *123*
Adrenergic system (ANS), 9–10
Aetiology
    acquired heart disease in cats, 34–38
    dilated cardiomyopathy
        (DCM), 26–27
    myxomatous mitral valve disease
        (MMVD), 16–18
Aldosterone, 9
Aldosterone antagonists, 109
American College of Veterinary Internal
        Medicine consensus statement
        (2019), 15, 19, 24, 33, 41, 43, 109
Angiotensin converting enzyme (ACE)
        inhibitors, 108

Angiotensin II, 9, **9**
Anticoagulants, 108
Antiplatelet drugs, 108
Antithrombotic therapy, 108
Aortic stenosis (AS), 52–53, *53*
Aortic thromboembolism (ATE), 37, **38**,
        43, 92, 119
    prognosis for, 47
Aortic valve, 4
Arrest rhythms, *79*, 79–80, *80*
Arrhythmias, 74–75
    collapse resulting from, 127–129, **128**
    drugs used in treatment of, 110–115
    treatment for, **128**
Artefact, **64**, 64–65, *65*
Asymptomatic CHD, 49–53
    aortic stenosis (AS), 52–53, *53*
    diseases causing left sided congestive
        heart failure (L-CHF), 49
    patent ductus arteriosus
        (PDA), 49–52
    ventricular septal defect (VSD), 49
Atrial fibrillation, 75–76, *76*
    clinical findings, 76
    ECG characteristics, 76
Atrial standstill, 79, *79*
    clinical findings, 79
    ECG characteristics, 79
Atrioventricular block, 77–79, *78*
    first degree, 77
    second degree, 77–78
    third degree, 78–79
Atrioventricular node (AV node), 8

Atrioventricular valves, 3–4
Audible arrythmias, 40–41
Auscultation, 39–41, 83–89
    heart murmur, 88–89, **89**, *89*
    stethoscope, 83, *84*
    technique, 84–86, *85–86*, **88**
    timing of additional heart sounds, 86, *87*

B

Beta adrenergic blockers, 114
Biomarkers, 46
Blood
    oxygenated, 6, *7*
    pathway of, 6
    sampling, 94–96, *95–96*
Blood pressure, 92–94
    equipment list, **93**
    how to take, 93–94
Bradyarrhythmias, 77–79, *79*
    atrial standstill, 79
    atrioventricular block, 77–79
    drugs used in management of, **116**
    treatment, 115
Bundle of His, 8

C

Cables, **60**, 60–61
Cardiac conduction system, *7*
    atrioventricular node (AV node), 8
    Bundle of His, 8
    Purkinje fibres, 8
    sinoatrial node (SA node), 7
Cardiac cycle, 6–7
    events of, 6
Cardiac emergencies, 119–129
    acute management of respiratory
        distress, 122–126
    after initial stabilisation, 120
    aims of, 119
    collapse, 119, 126–129
    feline aortic thromboembolism
        (FATE), 119
    initial client contact, 119
    life threatening arrythmias, 119

    presentation and emergency
        treatment, **121**
    respiratory distress, 119
Cardiomyopathy, 26, 33
Chambers of the heart, 4–6, *5*
Clinical signs
    of acquired heart disease in cats, 38–47
    dilated cardiomyopathy (DCM),
        27–28, **28**
    myxomatous mitral valve disease
        (MMVD), 18
    pericardial disease, 30
Clopidogrel, 108
Collapse, 119, 126–129
    resulting from arrythmia, 127–129, **128**
    resulting from severe
        disease, 126–127, *127*
Common arrythmias, 74–75
    common causes of, **75**
Compensated heart failure, 10
    cycle of, *10*
Compensatory mechanisms
    heart failure, 8–9, **9**
    myxomatous mitral valve disease
        (MMVD), 17–18, **18**
Conduction, *67*
Conduction system of the heart, 7–8
Congenital disease, 30, 49
Congenital heart disease
        (CHD), 49–57, **50**
    asymptomatic, 49–53
    cyanotic, 54–56
    right sided congestive heart failure
        (R-CHF), 53–54
Congestive heart failure (CHF), 105;
        see also Heart failure
    causes of, 12
    clinical signs associated with, **11**
Cyanotic CHD, 54–56
    Tetralogy of Fallot (ToF), 54–56, *56*

D

Decompensated heart failure, 10, 126
    cycle of, *11*

Diagnostic tests, 83–103
    dilated cardiomyopathy
        (DCM), 28–29
Diastolic dysfunction, 12
Digoxin, 107, 115
Dilated cardiomyopathy (DCM), 25–29,
        107
    aetiology, 26–27
    breeds with high prevalence of, **26**
    clinical signs, 27–28, **28**
    diagnostic tests, 28
    nursing and treatment of, 29
    prognosis, 28
    recommended diagnostic tests, 28–29
    signalment, 26
    staging of, 26, **26**
Diltiazem, 114
Diseases
    that cause left-sided CHF, 10, 49
    that cause right-sided CHF, 11
Diuretics, 105–107, **106**
    adverse effects of, 106
    furosemide, 105
    spironolactone, 106
    thiazides, 106
    torasemide, 105–106
Drugs
    antithrombotic drugs, 109–110
    natriuresis and diuresis, 105–107
    neurohormonal blockers, 108–109
    positive inotropes, 107–108
    used in treatment of arrhythmias,
        110–115
'Dub' sound, 83

E

Echocardiography, 100–102, *102*
Electrocardiograph (ECG) machine,
        59–65
    artefact, **64**, 64–65, *65*
    cables, **60**, 60–61
    electrodes, 59–60, **60**, *60*, **61**
    leads, 61–*63*
    settings, 64

Electrocardiography (ECGs), 1
    bradyarrhythmias, 77–79
    common arrythmias, 74–75
    interpretation, 67–73
    machine, 59–65
    positioning, 65–67
    sinus rhythms, 73–74
    tachyarrhythmias, 75–80
Electrodes, 59–60, **60**, *60*, **61**
European Society of Veterinary
        Cardiology, 28

F

Feline classification system, **41**
Feline heart disease, 108–109
    clinical signs of, **38**
    medications used in the treatment
        of, **111**
    nursing of, 41–47
    treatment of, 41–47
First degree AV block, 77
Forward heart failure, **12**, 12–13
Function of the heart, 3–13
Furosemide, 105

H

Heart
    cardiac cycle, 6–7
    causes of congestive heart
        failure, 12
    chambers of, 4–6, *5*
    conduction system of, 7–8
    forward failure, 12–13
    mechanisms of heart failure, 8–10
    pathway of blood, 6
    presentation of patients with heart
        failure, 10–12
    structure and function of, 3–13
Heart failure; *see also* Arrhythmias
    adrenergic system (ANS), 9–10
    compensatory mechanisms, 8–9, **9**
    congestive, **11**, 12, 105
    forward, **12**, 12–13

left sided congestive, 10, 49
mechanisms of, 8–10
medications used in treatment
    of, **111**
presentation of patients with, 10–12
renin-angiotensin-aldosterone system
    (RAAS), 8–9
right sided congestive, 11, 53–54, *54*
Heart murmur, 88–89, *89*
causes of, **89**
grading of, 88–89
Heart valves, 3–4
atrioventricular valves, 3–4
semilunar valves, 4
Heart wall, 3, *4*
Hypertrophic cardiomyopathy, 1, 13,
    33, **34**
Hypertrophic cardiomyopathy
    (HCM), 33, 34, *36*
breeds predisposed to, 34
on echocardiography, *36*

I

Interpretation
conduction system, *67*
electrocardiography, 67–73
guide, 68, **69**
P-QRS relationship, 69–73, *69–73*,
    71–72

L

Leads, 61–*63*
Left sided congestive heart failure
    (L-CHF), 10, 49
Lidocaine, 113
'lub' sound, 83

M

Mechanisms of heart failure, 8–10
Mexilitine, 114
Mitral valve, 3

Mitral valve disease, *see* Myxomatous
    mitral valve disease (MMVD)
Myocytes, **112**
Myxomatous mitral valve disease
    (MMVD), 15–25, 107, 126
aetiology, 16–18
alternative names for, 16
breeds predisposed to, 16
classification of, **20**
clinical signs, 18, 19
compensatory mechanisms, 17–18, **18**
nursing and treatment of, 19, **20**
nursing and treatment of stage A-D
    dogs, 20–25
prognosis, 18
signalment, 15–16

N

Natriuresis, 105–107
Neurohormonal blockers, **108**, 108–109
adverse effects of, 109
aldosterone antagonists, 109
angiotensin converting enzyme
    (ACE) inhibitors, 108
Nurse
auscultation, 83–89
blood pressure, 92–94
blood sampling, 94–96
echocardiography, 100–102
physical examination, 90–92
radiography, 96, 98–100
role in diagnostic tests, 83–103
Nursing
of dilated cardiomyopathy
    (DCM), 29
of feline heart disease, 41–47
of myxomatous mitral valve
    disease (MMVD), 19, **20**
of pericardial disease, 30

O

Oxygenated blood, 6, *7*

P

Patent ductus arteriosus (PDA), 49–52, *51, 52*
Pericardial disease, 30
  clinical signs, 30
  diagnosis, 30
  nursing and treatment of, 30
Pericardiocentesis, 124–126
  complications, 126
  kit, *125*
  preparing patient for, 124–126
Pharmacology, *see* Drugs
Phenotypes, 33, 34, **34**
Physical examination, 90–92, *90–92*, **91**
Pimobendan, 107
Positioning, of ECG machines, 65–67
  reasons for performing an ECG, 66
  tips for performing good quality
    ECG, 66–67
  troubleshooting guide, 66–67
Positive inotropes, **107**, 107–108
  adverse effects of, 107–108
  digoxin, 107
  nursing actions, 108
  pimobendan, 107
Pressure overload, 12
Prognosis
  of acquired heart disease in cats, 47
  for ATE, 47
  dilated cardiomyopathy (DCM), 28
  myxomatous mitral valve disease
    (MMVD), 18
Pulmonic stenosis (PS), 53–54, *54*
Pulmonic valve, 4
Purkinje fibres, 8

R

Radiography, 45–46, 96, *98*, 98–100, *99–101*
Renin-angiotensin aldosterone system
  (RAAS), 8–9
Right sided congestive heart failure
  (R-CHF), 53–54
  diseases causing, 11
  pulmonic stenosis (PS), 53–54, *54*

S

Second degree AV block, 77–78, *78*
  clinical findings, 78
  ECG characteristics, 77
Semilunar valves, 4
Signalment
  acquired heart disease in cats,
    33–34
  dilated cardiomyopathy (DCM), 26
  myxomatous mitral valve disease
    (MMVD), 15–16
Sinoatrial node (SA node), 7
Sinus arrythmia, 74, *74*
Sinus bradycardia, 74, *74*
Sinus rhythms, 73–74, *73–74*
  sinus arrythmia, 74, *74*
  sinus bradycardia, 74, *74*
  sinus tachycardia, 74, *74*
Sinus tachycardia, 74, *74*
Sotalol, 114
Spironolactone, 106
Stethoscope, 83, *84*
Structure of the heart, 3–13
Systolic anterior motion (SAM), 40, *40*
Systolic dysfunction, 12

T

Tachyarrhythmias, 75–80;
  see also Arrhythmias
  antiarrhythmic treatment
    of, 112–113, **113**
  arrest rhythms, *79*, 79–80, *80*
  atrial fibrillation, 75–76, *76*
  bradyarrhythmias, 77–79, *79*
  ventricular tachycardia, 76–77, *77*
Tetralogy of Fallot (ToF), 54–56, *56*
Thiazides, 106
Third degree AV block, 78–79, *78–79*
  clinical findings, 78–79
  ECG characteristics, 78
Thoracocentesis, 122–124, *123*
  kit, *122*
  preparing patient for, 122

Thromboembolism, 108–109
Torasemide, 105–106
Treatment
    of dilated cardiomyopathy
        (DCM), 29
    of feline heart disease, 41–47
    of myxomatous mitral valve disease
        (MMVD), 19, **20**
    of pericardial disease, 30
Tricuspid valve, 3

V

Vaughan-Williams classification,
    112–113, **113**
Venepuncture, *97*
Ventricular arrhythmias, 26–27
Ventricular septal defect (VSD), 49
Ventricular tachycardia, 76–77, *77*
    clinical findings, 76–77
    ECG characteristics, 76
Volume overload, 12

T - #0148 - 111024 - C162 - 229/152/7 - PB - 9780367641023 - Gloss Lamination